PREVENTION'S
Outsmart Diabetes

PREVENTION'S
Outsmart Diabetes

The Complete Easy-to-Use Plan
Plus 70 Delicious Recipes

By the Editors of PREVENTION. Magazine

RODALE

Notice

This book is intended as a reference volume only, not as a medical manual. The information given here is designed to help you make informed decisions about your health. It is not intended as a substitute for any treatment that may have been prescribed by your doctor. If you suspect that you have a medical problem, we urge you to seek competent medical help.

Mention of specific companies, organizations, or authorities in this book does not imply endorsement by the publisher, nor does mention of specific companies, organizations, or authorities in the book imply that they endorse the book.

Internet addresses and telephone numbers given in this book were accurate at the time this book went to press.

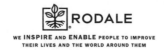

WE **INSPIRE** AND **ENABLE** PEOPLE TO IMPROVE
THEIR LIVES AND THE WORLD AROUND THEM

FOR PRODUCTS & INFORMATION
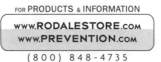

(800) 848-4735

Contents

PART **ONE**

Diabetes Explained

From what it is to how it's treated, find out
everything you need to know about this disease

Understanding what's happening is
the first step to taking control

Diabetes medications and how they work,
plus the promise the future holds

From basic monitors to the newest tracking tests,
here's what you need to know

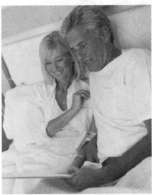

Medications
Know all
your options.
p. 10

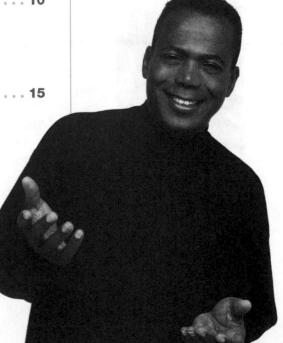

A Diabetes Primer
Get the answers that
will put you in control.
p. 2

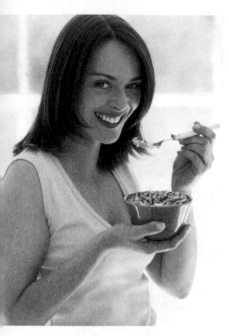

Prevent Early Diabetes
Fiber-rich whole grains
help control blood sugar.
p. 22

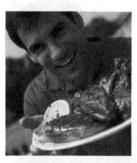

**Know the
Exchange System**
Devise the perfect
food plan for you.
p. 38

PART **TWO**

Stop Diabetes Before It Starts

Take control, and prevent "early diabetes"
from developing into the full-fledged disease

PART **THREE**

Eat to Beat Diabetes

Take control of this disease by simply
choosing more of the right foods

PART **FOUR**
Exercise Prescriptions for Diabetes

Get moving—even just a little bit—and
watch your blood sugar improve

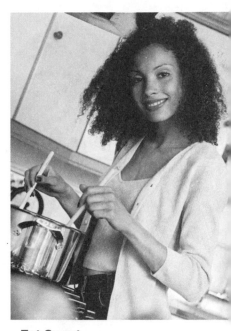

Eat Smart
Improve your blood
sugar by 95%!
p. 38

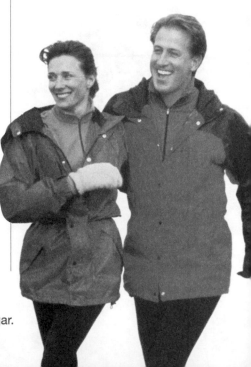

Walk It Down
Just three times a week lowers blood sugar.
p. 70

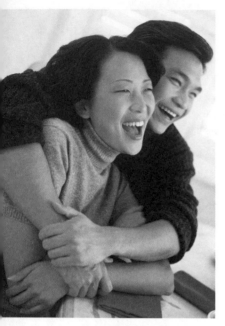

Feel Good!
Regular checkups
will keep you well.
p. 92

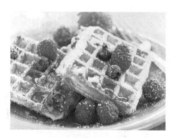

Rich Vanilla Waffles
Low-fat, calcium-rich,
and delicious!
p. 111

CHAPTER **19**

Whip up a quick soup, salad, or sandwich from
this collection of 10 healing recipes

CHAPTER **20**

Choose from 27 delicious dinners that will satisfy
your tastebuds *and* take care of your body

CHAPTER **21**

Craving an after-dinner indulgence? Here are 16
mouthwatering treats that won't derail your blood sugar

CHAPTER **22**

These nine snacks and sweets aren't just tasty—
they're good for you too

Chocolate Malted Shake
Creamy, refreshing,
and low in fat.
p. 174

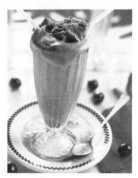

Shop Smart
Buy the right foods to
control diabetes.
p. 178

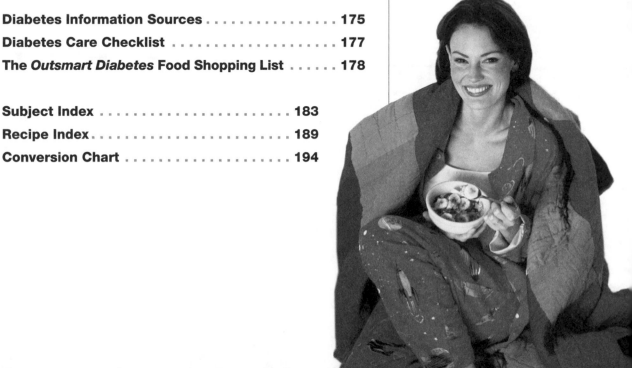

INTRODUCTION
Get Control of Your Life Again!

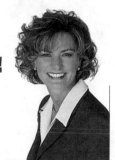

Gone are the days when a diagnosis of diabetes meant a lifetime of misery. With a deeper understanding of how this condition works, we now know that a healthier lifestyle gives you control over your diabetes and lowers your chance of developing complications. And that leads to a longer, more enjoyable life.

That's why we've put together this special book for you. We've gathered the latest information from the nation's top diabetes experts and combined it with *Prevention*'s commitment to excellence and good health to bring you a comprehensive diabetes guide you can trust.

This book will tell you how to get tested and what to do to keep early diabetes from becoming something worse. You'll discover the most important things you can do to get your blood sugar under control: Eat smart (p. 38), exercise regularly (p. 68), understand how your medications work (p. 10), and lose weight if you're overweight (p. 84).

You'll also discover the best blood sugar tests on the market today and what's in the works (p. 15), how to enjoy dining at restaurants (p. 56), how to prevent diabetes-related complications (p. 92), and so much more.

You'll also find a special recipe section featuring 70 delicious comfort foods that are so good, your whole family will love them. You can enjoy favorites such as macaroni and cheese, chicken potpie, even chocolaty brownies without worrying that you're sending your blood sugar out of control.

I urge you to read this book carefully, get yourself tested, and do whatever it takes to pull the reins in on this disease. And, as always, please let us know what we can do to help.

Catherine M. Cassidy

Catherine Cassidy
Editor-in-Chief
Prevention magazine

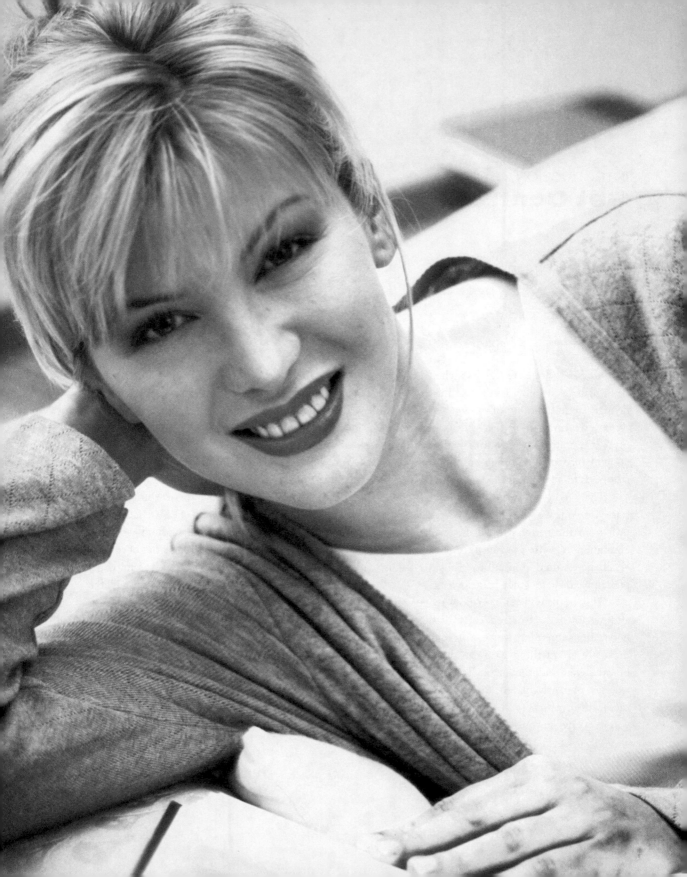

Diabetes Explained

From what it is to how it's treated, find out everything you need to know about this disease

CHAPTER 1

All Your Diabetes Questions Answered

Understanding what's happening is the first step to taking control

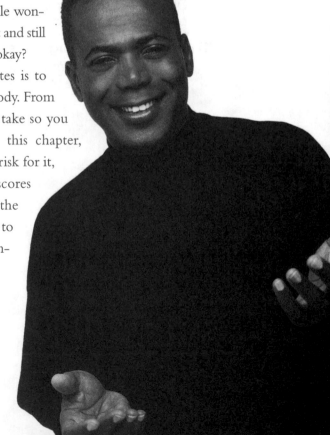

Although approximately 2,200 people are diagnosed with diabetes each day, the cause of this condition still remains a mystery. People wonder: What is this disease? How can I have it and still feel fine? What's the treatment? Will I be okay?

The first step to outsmarting diabetes is to understand what is happening in your body. From there, you'll learn exactly what steps to take so you can enjoy a long and healthy life. In this chapter, you'll find out what diabetes is, who's at risk for it, when to get tested (and what the test scores mean), and more. Once you have all the facts, you'll find that *you* have the power to control diabetes—instead of it having control over you!

What Is Diabetes?

When you have diabetes, something is wrong with your production of insulin, a vital hormone made by your pancreas. Insulin helps your cells take in fuel in the form of blood sugar. (This blood sugar, also called glucose, is produced when your body digests food.) If glucose doesn't get into the cells, they begin to weaken. Then the sugar from your food builds up in the blood-stream, damaging everything from your blood vessels to your organs.

Although both type 1 and type 2 diabetes deal with insulin, they work differently. In type 1 diabetes, the pancreas either no longer produces insulin, or it doesn't produce enough of it. In type 2 diabetes, your pancreas makes insulin, but the body isn't able to use it properly.

TAKE CONTROL: Know the Symptoms

Diabetes has a host of symptoms, many of which you may never have thought were associated with the disease. If you have any of these 12 symptoms, ask your doctor to test you for diabetes.

▶ Frequent urination

▶ Excessive thirst

▶ Unexplained weight loss

▶ Unusual hunger

▶ Extreme fatigue

▶ Irritability

▶ Frequent infections

▶ Blurred vision

▶ Slow-to-heal cuts and bruises

▶ Vaginitis or recurring yeast infections in women

▶ Tingling or numbness in the hands or feet

▶ Recurring skin, gum, or bladder infections

Why Does It Go Unnoticed?

Unlike many other diseases, diabetes isn't obvious. Often you feel just fine. And its complications can mask themselves as other health problems first. It hides behind cardiovascular disease, kidney disease, nerve damage, and eye disease. "Most of the diagnoses are delayed by an average of 7 years. So by the time people know they have it, it's firmly established and difficult to treat. And long-term complications have already gained a foothold," says Harvard researcher David M. Nathan, MD, director of the diabetes center at Massachusetts General Hospital and chairman of the huge National Institutes of Health Diabetes Prevention Program. Of the nearly 16 million people with diabetes, only one-third realize they have it.

Is It Curable?

Neither form of diabetes is curable. But with the right treatment, you can get your blood sugar back down to normal. As long as you keep your glucose levels at an acceptable level, you should be able to live a normal and healthy life.

Who Is at Risk?

Type 1 diabetes, sometimes referred to as juvenile or insulin-dependent diabetes, often occurs in people younger than 30 who are not overweight. Type 2 diabetes, formerly known as adult-onset diabetes, typically develops in people over 30 who have one or more risk factors for the disease. (See "Are You at Risk?" on p. 6 for more on risk factors.)

The Invisible Threat

Early diabetes—having higher-than-normal blood sugar levels—has no symptoms that you or your doctor can feel or see. But it's a silent threat. Here's why you can't ignore it.

What Happens to You

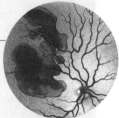

Half of the 20 to 30 million Americans with early diabetes will have full-blown type 2 diabetes within 10 years. This raises their risk for serious complications, including blindness, kidney failure, and possible bone fractures.

Broken blood vessels in the eye

How You Get It

Overweight and high stress can make your body store fat around internal organs. This visceral fat is linked to extra fat storage in the liver—which can raise blood sugar levels— and to extra fat in muscle cells, making them resist insulin. Physical inactivity also creates insulin resistance. The result is a dangerous rise in blood sugar levels.

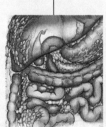

Visceral fat around internal organs

Early diabetes also raises your risk for heart disease, high blood pressure, and stroke. It is linked to the thickening of artery walls and to a lethal kind of cholesterol called small, dense LDLs, which cause dangerous clogs and clots.

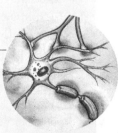

Blood clot

Full-blown type 2 diabetes raises the odds of nerve damage throughout the body, which can lead to pain, numbness, and even amputation. Early diabetes increases the chances you'll get type 2 diabetes and, eventually, damaged nerves.

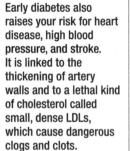

Nerve damage

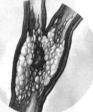
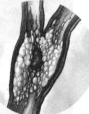
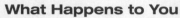

But know this: Being at risk for diabetes does not mean you're destined to develop the disease. What it does mean is that you need to be extravigilant about watching out for symptoms and getting yourself tested on a regular basis.

How Can I Lower My Child's Risk?

When most people think of children and diabetes, they think of type 1. Though experts have some theories, the cause of type 1 diabetes is still unknown, says Marian Parrott, MD, vice president of clinical affairs at the American Diabetes Association (ADA). In fact, 90% of children with type 1 diabetes have no family history of the disease. What we do know is that the body doesn't produce enough insulin, so insulin shots are needed to control blood sugar levels. (See "All about Insulin" on p. 11 for more on this treatment.)

Until experts pinpoint the cause of type 1 diabetes, there's not much parents can do to prevent it. However, type 2 diabetes is on the rise among children, and this form of childhood diabetes is very preventable. Here's how to lower your child's chances of getting the disease.

Know the risk factors. Type 2 diabetes in children is strongly linked to a family history of the disease. If you had diabetes while pregnant,

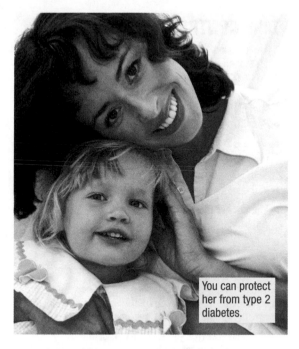

You can protect her from type 2 diabetes.

your child may be at increased risk for diabetes later in life, so you may want to have a discussion with your doctor about having her tested. While approximately 36% of children whose mothers had gestational diabetes are obese and have impaired glucose tolerance, it's unclear how much is genetic and how much is due to being exposed to higher glucose levels when in the uterus. To reduce your risk of developing gestational diabetes in future pregnancies, see "Diabetes during Pregnancy" on p. 9.

Watch her weight. A healthy lifestyle is as important for children as adults, especially since

Being at risk for diabetes does not mean you're destined to develop it. What it does mean is that you should be tested so you can take action quickly if you get it.

TAKE CONTROL: Are You at Risk?

If you have any of the following risk factors, you may be at increased risk of developing diabetes. While everyone must be on the watch for diabetes, you need to be particularly vigilant about watching for symptoms and getting tested.

▶ You have a family history of diabetes.

▶ You are 20% over a healthy weight, or obese. (Your doctor can tell you whether or not you're in this category.)

▶ You lead a sedentary lifestyle.

▶ You are African-American, Latino, Asian, Native American, or a Pacific Islander.

▶ You had diabetes during pregnancy or had a baby who was 9 lb or more at birth. (See "Diabetes during Pregnancy" on p. 9 for more on gestational diabetes.)

▶ You are 45 or older. (While it's wise to be tested as early as age 25 if you're at risk, the older you are, the greater your risk becomes.)

▶ You have low HDL (good) cholesterol or high overall cholesterol levels.

▶ You have very high blood pressure or very high triglycerides.

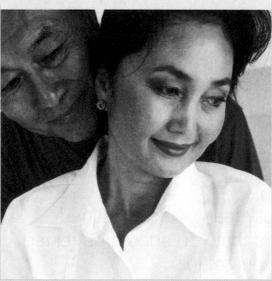

obesity may be a risk factor for childhood type 2 diabetes. Feed your child a healthy, balanced diet that's low in fat. Encourage activity by limiting sedentary pursuits, including time in front of the TV and computer.

When Should I Get Tested?

Even if you have no symptoms, don't put off getting tested. "Diabetes is like lead paint in houses with little kids," says Gerald Bernstein, MD, former president of the ADA. Symptoms don't appear until the damage is done. By the time diabetes is nabbed, 20% of patients are having vision or cardiovascular problems.

Besides, only one-third of the people who wind up with a diagnosis actually develop—and notice—the classic symptoms. So when should you get tested? If you have any of the risk factors and symptoms of diabetes and you are younger than 45, you should discuss getting tested with your doctor. According to a study from the Centers for Disease Control and Prevention (CDC) in Atlanta, testing before age 45 can uncover the condition 5 to 6 years earlier than it would otherwise be detected.

As for regular testing, experts recommend that people over 45 be considered for testing every year if they have any risk factors, and every 3 years if they don't. The earlier you can detect diabetes, the more time you have to treat it and avoid diabetes-related complications. Further review is needed before experts will recommend testing for all Americans before age 45, says lead study researcher Michael Engelgau, MD.

The Best Time to Test for Diabetes

When researchers from the National Institute of Diabetes and Digestive and Kidney Diseases (NIDDK) reviewed results of fasting plasma glucose tests given to 12,800 adults, they found that afternoon tests showed significantly lower blood glucose levels than morning tests. In fact, the levels were low enough that only half of the afternoon test subjects expected to have diabetes would have actually qualified as diabetic by current standards.

If you're scheduled for a diabetes check, ask for a morning appointment. Or discuss with your doctor the researchers' suggestion that afternoon test results may indicate diabetes at glucose levels of 114 mg/dl or higher, instead of the standard 126 mg/dl.

What Do I Need to Know about Testing?

The ADA recommends the fasting plasma glucose (FPG) test for your first screening. It measures blood sugar levels and is inexpensive, at just $5 to $10. (Sometimes insurance may even cover it.) This test can be done by your family doctor or by a testing laboratory.

You have to fast (that is, consume no food or drink other than water) for at least 8 hours before the FPG test. To minimize hunger pains, schedule the test early in the morning so you can fast mostly in your sleep. After you fast, your doctor or a lab technician draws a sample of your blood, and the amount of glucose in the blood is measured.

What Do the Test Scores Mean?

If the FPG test measures blood sugar at **126 mg/dl or higher,** you have diabetes. A diagnosis of diabetes is made when two diagnostic

tests done on different days show that your blood glucose level is too high. The ADA previously defined diabetes as anything higher than 140 mg/dl, but they recently lowered the number to 126 mg/dl to encourage people to begin treating diabetes sooner, thereby preventing complications.

If blood sugar is **between 110 and 125 mg/dl,** it indicates "troubled blood sugar"—a category newly identified by the ADA and known as impaired fasting glucose (IFG). Consider this a warning: You could be on your way to diabetes. But the good news is that you can take steps to try to avoid developing a full-blown case.

What Can Happen If I Don't Control My Blood Sugar?

We've already mentioned the long-term complications that can arise from not taking care of your diabetes. But there are also immediate problems

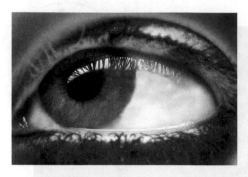

Eye Scan Tests for Diabetes

Your eye doctor may soon be able to check for early signs of uncontrolled blood sugar levels and type 2 diabetes. The device used, the Accu-Chek D-Tector, measures certain compounds that build up more quickly in the eyes of those with high blood sugar levels than in the eyes of those with normal levels.

The eye scan takes less than 30 seconds, and abnormal results would have to be followed by more specific tests. It is just finishing FDA-required final clinical trials. If all goes well, it could reach the market this year, says Donna Whipple, global marketing director at Roche Diagnostics in Indianapolis, one of the companies developing the device.

that can occur when your blood sugar spikes too high or drops too low.

High blood sugar (also known as hyperglycemia). Your blood sugar may go too high if you don't take care of your condition, or when you are sick or under a lot of stress. Symptoms of high blood sugar include headaches, blurred vision, thirst, frequent urination, and dry, itchy skin. Drink lots of water when you are sick or have high blood sugar, and use medication and lifestyle changes to get it back down.

Low blood sugar (also known as hypoglycemia). It is possible to have too little glucose in your system. This can be caused by taking too much diabetes medicine, eating too little or not eating at all, exercising too hard or too long, and drinking alcohol without eating. When blood sugar drops, you feel shaky, tired, hungry, confused, and nervous.

What's the Next Step?

Once you are diagnosed, you and your doctor will discuss lifestyle changes and possible medications that you may have to take. But as we've said before, diabetes and your health are totally under your control. By doing the right things (which you'll find throughout this book), you'll live a long, happy, healthy life!

TAKE CONTROL: Have Your Kids Tested Too

Even though Leslie Wiles had worked as a nurse for more than 25 years, it was her "mother's intuition," not her medical training, that led to a diabetes diagnosis for her 7-year-old daughter, Alex. Now, thanks to treatment, Alex has learned how to modify her life to keep her blood sugar under control. If you suspect that your child has diabetes, have her physician test her as soon as possible so you can begin to treat it.

Diabetes during Pregnancy

By definition, gestational diabetes appears only in pregnant women who haven't previously had either type 1 or type 2 diabetes, or about 2 to 5% of pregnancies. After the pregnancy ends, so does the diabetes. The risk factors are the same for gestational diabetes as for type 2 diabetes. But even women with none of the risk factors can develop gestational diabetes, which is why pregnant women who are at risk (those over the age of 25 or those under 25 and obese) are screened with an oral glucose tolerance test between the 24th and 28th weeks of pregnancy. Here's what gestational diabetes means for your baby and you.

Your baby: Fortunately, by the time gestational diabetes is detected, a baby's organs are already fully formed, and the baby won't develop diabetes. In time, however, the extra blood sugar can cross back through the placenta, causing problems for the fetus such as hypoglycemia (low blood sugar). Although rare, the risk of birth defects is slightly higher in babies born to moms with diabetes.

One of the biggest problems of gestational diabetes is that the babies are large. It's called macrosomia, and while big babies can be healthy babies, they are difficult to deliver and may be injured during the delivery. This is one reason that doctors may choose to induce early labor or recommend a cesarean section in mothers who develop gestational diabetes.

You: If you develop gestational diabetes, here's what you need to do.

➤ Have your glucose levels monitored closely throughout the pregnancy.

➤ Get nutritional counseling so that you'll be eating properly to meet the needs of pregnancy.

➤ Talk to your doctor about medication. Although oral medications for diabetes have not been recommended for pregnant women in the past, a new study of oral glyburide showed no significant difference in the health of the mothers compared with injected insulin. Also, the babies weighed the same and showed the same blood sugar levels at birth.

➤ Get tested at your 6-week postdelivery checkup to make sure you don't develop type 2 diabetes later. If the tests are normal, it's recommended that you be tested for diabetes every 3 years, since gestational diabetes is a risk factor for type 2 diabetes.

➤ Be on the alert for gestational diabetes in future pregnancies.

➤ To lower your risk, follow a healthy diet, start a postbaby exercise regimen as soon as your doctor

CHAPTER 2

What You Need to Know about Medications

Diabetes medications and how they work, plus the promise the future holds

Although a healthy diet and an active lifestyle are important parts of managing diabetes, some people need extra help in the form of prescription drugs or insulin to keep their blood sugar under control. As you take responsibility for your health, it's important to understand how the various diabetes medications work. For instance, there are many medications for type 2 diabetes, and each works slightly differently. There are also different ways to administer insulin. Here you'll learn all about the various types of oral diabetes medications and insulin and how they work—all explained in easy-to-understand language, not medical jargon. When you know all your options, you and your doctor can work together to find the best treatment plan for you.

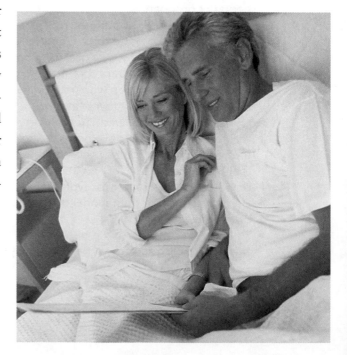

Why Is Medication Necessary?

In type 1 diabetes, the pancreas doesn't produce enough (or any) insulin, a hormone that escorts blood sugar—also known as glucose—throughout the body. Without enough insulin, all that sugar builds up and damages blood vessels and other parts of your body. That's why if you have type 1 diabetes, you need to supplement your body with insulin to help keep your blood sugar under control.

In type 2 diabetes, you make insulin, but your body becomes resistant to it. So you need to take oral medications that help keep those blood sugar levels in check. Eventually you may need to take insulin as well. That's because your body's needs may change over time, so diet and exercise alone may not always be enough to keep blood sugar in check.

All about Insulin

If your doctor determines that the best way to control your diabetes is by taking insulin, you have several choices. In fact, not only are there different kinds of insulin available, but there are also different methods of getting it into your body. (The chart on p. 14 lists the four main categories of insulin currently available.) Here's what you need to know.

Where it comes from. Among the more than 20 types of insulin sold in the US, some is produced by pigs or cows. Other insulin is manufactured in laboratories so that it is identical to human insulin.

How it's delivered. As of now, insulin cannot be taken as a pill, because it would

On the Horizon: Insulin Injection Alternatives

Experts are researching methods of insulin delivery that don't require needles at all. Here's what they're working on.

Insulin pills. Until now, insulin pills have been ineffective, because stomach enzymes break down the insulin before it has a chance to work. But researchers at Purdue University in West Lafayette, IN, have created a gel-like substance that protects insulin until it gets into the small intestine. At that point, the insulin can be absorbed into the bloodstream. This method has yet to be tested in humans, but preliminary studies in the lab and in animals are encouraging.

Insulin inhalers. To bypass the problem of stomach acids breaking down insulin, the medicine is sprayed directly into the mouth as a mist. It coats the throat, tongue, and the rest of the mouth, where it can pass through the membranes and directly into the bloodstream. Diabetic patients are now being tested, and so far the inhaler is performing well. Both type 1 and type 2 diabetics can use it, but type 1 still would require insulin shots. The insulin inhaler should be available soon.

be broken down during digestion just like protein in food. It must be injected for it to get into your bloodstream. There are several ways to deliver insulin.

Insulin syringes. You fill a syringe from a bottle and inject it as directed by your physician. You can purchase more than one bottle at a time,

---

TAKE CONTROL: Stay with the Program

Even if you're currently taking diabetes medications, eating right and exercising regularly will not only help you control your diabetes, but it could affect the performance of those medications, diminish your need for them, and possibly help keep you off insulin even longer.

---

but extras must be refrigerated until you're ready to use them.

Insulin pens. These handy devices come in either disposable or refillable form. Some people find pens easier to use, because they don't have to carry around bottles and needles. However, the cartridges of insulin pens contain only one type of insulin, so you have to make two injections if you're using two types of insulin.

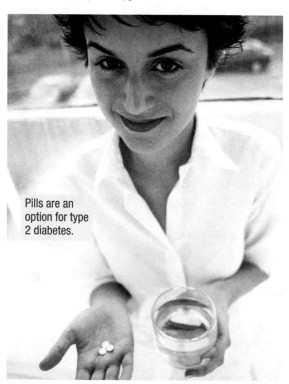

Pills are an option for type 2 diabetes.

Insulin pumps. The insulin pump, which may be as small as a beeper, is worn on your belt or in your clothes. It delivers insulin through a thin tube to a special needle inserted in the skin. The unit contains a battery-operated pump, an insulin reservoir, and a tiny computer that you program with dosage information. Because these pumps provide a tighter control on insulin levels, many people who use them believe they're able to enjoy a more flexible lifestyle.

‖ Oral Medications

Today there are many oral medications for the treatment of type 2 diabetes, but that hasn't always been the case. Until the mid-1980s, there was only insulin and one class of oral medication called the sulfonylureas. But thanks to advances in research, several new types of oral medications have been developed over the past 5 years, giving doctors and patients more options for better controlling type 2 diabetes. Note: Depending on the medication and how it works, you may need to eat according to a certain schedule to maximize the drug's effectiveness. Discuss this and any other lifestyle requirements with your doctor before you start taking these medications.

Sulfonylureas (Chlorpropamide, Acetazolamide, Tolazamide, Glyburide, and Glipizide) lower blood glucose by causing the pancreas to

Secret Prescription Help

Here's some good news: You can get medications for free, or nearly free, if you meet criteria set by pharmaceutical companies—even, in some cases, if you earn more than $50,000 annually. You may qualify if . . .

➤ You don't have outpatient prescription drug coverage and aren't covered by any government programs that pay for drugs.

➤ You can prove that buying a high-priced drug would cause you financial hardship.

➤ You've exceeded prescription drug coverage limits set by your insurance company (applicable in some cases).

These programs most often help middle-income adults in times of sudden major illness. The programs can also help when the cost of treating a chronic condition is high. But they are so underpublicized that doctors aren't always aware that they exist.

Most major pharmaceutical companies have a program. Some require physicians to contact them, while others allow patients to apply directly. An organization called The Medicine Program contacts drug manufacturers on behalf of patients. "All kinds of medications, from diabetes drugs to cancer drugs to long-term prescriptions for insulin, arthritis, cholesterol, and hormone replacement therapies, are covered," says Cindy Hogg, cofounder of The Medicine Program.

Talk to your doctor, or contact The Medicine Program directly at (573) 996-7300. You can also visit their Web site at www.themedicineprogram.com for an application and brochure.

release more insulin. While these drugs are effective in many patients, they don't work for everyone, so you may have to switch to insulin or other oral medications at some point. If you take sulfonylureas, you'll need to pay particular attention to eating on schedule to avoid low blood sugar reactions.

Nateglinide (Starlix) is a new type of diabetes drug recently approved by the FDA that could help prevent dangerous episodes of low blood sugar in people with type 2 diabetes. Starlix stimulates the pancreas to produce insulin quickly, then "turns itself off" before too much reaches the bloodstream. (Too-high insulin levels are a side effect of some other diabetes medica-

tions, prompting the body's cells to take up too much sugar from the blood.) Starlix also helps control postmeal rises in blood sugar.

Meglitinide (Repaglinide) works much like sulfonylureas to increase production of insulin by the pancreas, but it's shorter acting.

TAKE CONTROL: Warm Your Insulin

Injecting cold insulin can make shots more painful. To make things easier on yourself, let the bottle that's currently in use set out until it reaches room temperature, or gently roll the cold bottle between your hands to heat it up. Don't put insulin in direct sunlight or in the freezer; extreme temperatures can destroy the hormone.

TAKE CONTROL: Ask about Long-Acting Insulin

Lantus, one of the most recent injectable diabetes medications, provides a consistent insulin supply for 24 hours. It may prove convenient for those with type 1 diabetes who currently need three or four insulin injections a day, as well as those with type 2 diabetes who require both insulin injections and oral medications. Its smooth, predictable effect on blood sugar levels helps minimize the risk of low blood sugar reactions. Consult your doctor if you're interested in exploring this option.

Biguanide (Metformin) decreases the liver's production of glucose and also improves the effectiveness of the insulin secreted by the pancreas. Proper bloodflow to the kidneys is required to take this medication, so your heart and kidney function, as well as your age, will determine whether or not you can take this drug.

Alpha-glycosides inhibitors (Acarbose and Meglitol) delay the digestion of sugars and starches from the intestines, which leads to lower blood sugar after meals. Because these drugs work in the gastrointestinal tract instead of the bloodstream, they can cause side effects such as bloating and gas.

Thiazolidinediones (Rosiglitazone and Pioglitazone) don't work on the pancreas. Instead, this class of drugs increases the effectiveness of the insulin that's released. Liver problems can be a side effect of thiazolidinediones, but with liver monitoring and improvements in these drugs, the problems have been reduced.

Insulin in Action

If you're taking insulin, here's a handy reference that shows how fast and how long each type works.

Type of Insulin	Starts Working	Peak Action	Duration of Action
RAPID-ACTING (Insulin Lispro)	Within 15 minutes	30–90 minutes	Less than 5 hours
SHORT-ACTING (Regular)	In ½–1 hour	2–4 hours	6–8 hours
INTERMEDIATE-ACTING (NPH, Lente)	In 1–4 hours	6–10 hours	10–16 hours
LONG-ACTING (Ultralente)	In 4–6 hours	18 hours	24–36 hours

CHAPTER 3

The Best Blood Sugar Tests

From basic monitors to the newest tracking tests, here's what you need to know

If you have diabetes, you know that monitoring your blood glucose levels helps reduce your risk of disease-related complications. In addition to the tried-and-true blood glucose monitor, researchers have come up with other devices that can help you keep track of your blood sugar ups and downs and enable your doctor to fine-tune your treatment. This type of tracking helps to identify your body's unique blood sugar trends so that your medication can be tailored to your particular needs—thus treating your diabetes as effectively as possible. In this chapter you'll also learn about a potentially lifesaving test that many people with diabetes don't get. Here's everything you need to know about the testing devices that will enable you to take charge of your health—and happiness!

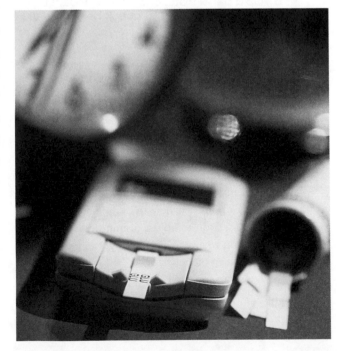

A Diabetes Care Checklist

When researchers from the Centers for Disease Control and Prevention (CDC) in Atlanta analyzed survey data from about 15,000 people with diabetes, they found a surprising health care gap: Fewer than 45% checked their blood sugar levels daily, fewer than 60% got an annual eye exam or foot exam, and fewer than 25% had an annual HbA1c test, which helps determine whether blood sugar is under control.

"People with diabetes have an increased risk for heart disease as well as other complications that affect the eyes, kidneys, and feet," says lead researcher Stephanie Benjamin, PhD, epidemiologist with the CDC. The best protection? Regular checks can help diabetics live a longer and better life, she says.

Must-Have Monitoring

If you have diabetes, get these five checks regularly:

Test	How Often
1. Blood sugar self-monitoring (as directed by your doctor)	Daily
2. Blood test for glycated hemoglobin (HbA1c)	At least once a year
3. Foot check for sores or ulcers (performed by your physician)	At least once a year
4. Eye screening for retinopathy, a condition that can lead to blindness	Once a year
5. Lipid panel (total cholesterol, HDL, LDL, and triglycerides) to check heart disease risk	Once a year

Blood Sugar Testing Essential

The Blood Glucose Monitor

For people with diabetes, self-monitoring of blood glucose levels can be vital to reducing complications related to the disease. Blood glucose monitors for home use help to oversee drug therapy and allow you to adjust insulin doses. They also alert you to any needed changes in exercise or diet between office visits.

To use a monitor, you apply blood from a finger prick to a chemically active test strip. Then place the strip in a meter that analyzes and displays your glucose level. Depending on the type and severity of your diabetes, you may need to check your blood sugar several times a day.

Monitors vary in terms of price and features. The more expensive ones display results in chart or graph form and download results to computer software. But whether you purchase a simple monitor or one with many features, the results are generally accurate, says Bruce R. Zimmerman, MD, former president of the American Diabetes Association (ADA). Costs range from $34 to $115 for the monitoring kit (onetime purchase) and from $65 to $70 for 100 disposable strips. If you have a monitor that's more than 5 years old, however, think about replacing it for newer technology, advises Dr. Zimmerman. There's no prescription required, but Medicare and some insurers require one for reimbursement.

Tracking Blood Sugar Trends

The MiniMed Continuous Glucose Monitoring System

The MiniMed Continuous Glucose Monitoring System is a pager-size unit equipped with a tiny sensor. Inserted under the skin, the sensor measures blood glucose levels every 5 minutes for 2 to 3 days. "The difference between this and a finger-stick test is like the difference between a movie and a still photograph," says Alan Marcus, MD, of the University of Southern California School of Medicine in Los Angeles. "Once the physician knows how glucose levels rise and fall throughout the day, he can refine therapy so that levels are always in a safe range."

This device will supplement, rather than replace, the finger-stick blood glucose self-tests that patients now perform. The unit is FDA-approved for type 1 diabetes; researchers are studying whether it can also be used for type 2.

TAKE CONTROL: Get Your Shot
Diabetes increases the risk of respiratory infection, so get a pneumococcal vaccine and a yearly flu shot.

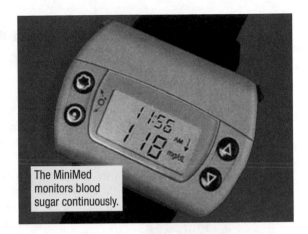
The MiniMed monitors blood sugar continuously.

Needle-Free Blood Sugar Monitoring

The GlucoWatch Biographer

Now you can use a watchlike device to help keep track of your blood sugar ups and downs. The GlucoWatch Biographer is a noninvasive monitor that provides continuous glucose readings without the traditional pricking and bleeding.

Developed and manufactured by Cygnus, GlucoWatch uses low-level electrical current to pull glucose (rather than blood) through the skin for measurement—a process known as reverse iontophoresis. It can provide glucose readings up to three times an hour, day or night, for up to 12 hours at a stretch. It also creates an electronic diary of up to 4,000 glucose readings, so you can detect trends and track patterns in your glucose levels over time, which can come in handy when you and your doctor are planning diet, exercise, and medication schedules. The downside: Gluco-Watch does not replace traditional finger-stick glucose checks, because its results may be inaccurate about one-quarter of the time.

The Test You Need—And May Not Be Getting

What it is: The hemoglobin A1c test (also known as the HbA1c or glycated hemoglobin test) gives a long-range blood sugar picture that shows how well blood glucose has been controlled over a period of up to 3 months. It doesn't replace the "snapshots" of daily blood sugar monitoring, but rather gives a picture over time. Both views are important, says Terry Maratos-Flier, MD, associate professor of medicine at Harvard University Medical School and head of the obesity section at the Joslin Diabetes Center in Boston.

How it works: Hemoglobin, a protein in the red blood cells, ferries oxygen to the body's cells. While it's busy delivering oxygen, the hemoglobin also picks up—

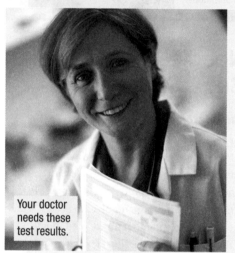

Your doctor needs these test results.

or "glycates" itself with—glucose. Most of the attached glucose is in a form called hemoglobin A1c. The more glucose in the blood, the more A1c there is.

Why it's important: This new test tells your doctor whether your diabetes is really under control or if you're having too many high-sugar spikes. It's potentially helpful for women contemplating pregnancy to assure that their blood sugar has been under control over a period of time, which is vital for having a healthy pregnancy and a healthy baby. (High blood sugar can lead to problems for mother and baby; see chapter 1.)

Interpreting test results:
An HbA1c level at or below 6% is normal.
An HbA1c level of 7% corresponds to a blood sugar level over time of about 150 (elevated blood sugar).
An HbA1c level of 8% corresponds to a blood sugar level over time of about 180.

Studies show that the average HbA1c level for type 2 diabetics in the US is 9.4%, which corresponds to a blood sugar level of 220. The American Diabetes Association recommends taking action when levels get to 8% and recommends a goal of less than 7%. Research shows that when the HbA1c level is kept below 7%, there's less risk of complications to organs such as the kidneys, eyes, and nerves.

How often should you be tested?
Up to four times a year at most if you have type 1 or type 2 diabetes and use insulin.
Twice a year if you have type 2 and don't use insulin.
Every 2 weeks if your diabetes has been way out of control and you're now trying to correct it.
If you're pregnant and have diabetes, have your HbA1c measured every 1 to 2 months to tell if your blood sugar is staying under control.

Available by prescription only, GlucoWatch costs about $450 and uses sensor pads costing about $5 that must be changed daily. For more information, call toll-free (866) 459-2824, or visit the manufacturer's Web site at www.glucowatch .com.

Tracking Trends in the Future

The Diasensor 2000

A new clinical study will test a device called the Diasensor 2000, which works by beaming an infrared light painlessly through the skin's surface to measure blood sugar. While it won't replace the finger-prick test completely, it's a tool that, like the MiniMed and GlucoWatch, could be helpful in gauging overall blood sugar trends.

"Finding the trends in blood glucose levels is extremely important," says Francesco Celi, MD, a diabetes specialist at the University of Maryland Joslin Diabetes Center in Baltimore and clinical coordinator of the study. "The Diasensor 2000 is useful for giving us averages at different times, and we can then decide how to treat the patient." If approved in the US, the Diasensor 2000 would be individually calibrated for each patient and used in the home under medical supervision.

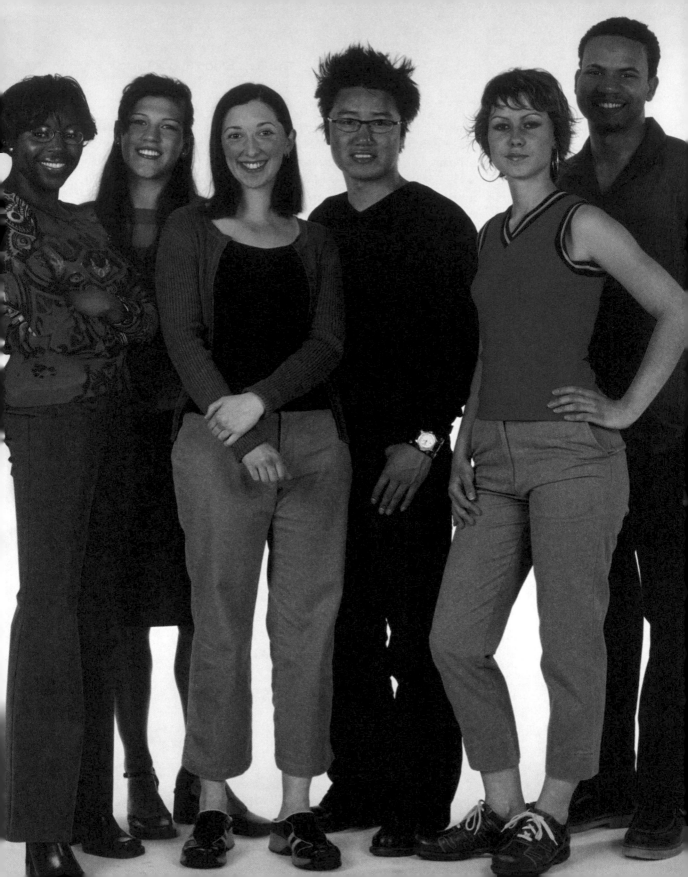

PART **TWO**

Stop Diabetes Before It Starts

Take control, and prevent "early diabetes" from developing into the full-fledged disease

CHAPTER 4

Block Diabetes with Food and Fitness

Stop diabetes in its tracks with lifestyle changes that are proven to work

An estimated 20 to 30 million Americans have early diabetes—often referred to as impaired glucose tolerance—and don't even know it. This is a symptomless condition in which blood sugar rises higher than normal, enough to put you at risk of serious complications but not quite high enough to fit current definitions of type 2 diabetes.

But the good news is that you can keep impaired glucose tolerance from developing into full-blown diabetes simply by changing the way you eat and getting a little bit of exercise. For instance, adding more fiber-rich, low-fat whole grains, fruits, and vegetables to your diet and going for walks several times a week can make a big difference in your blood sugar levels. Here's all you need to know— and exactly what you can do to ward off diabetes.

Defining Early Diabetes

In 2000, the Centers for Disease Control and Prevention (CDC) in Atlanta made headlines with the shocking news that type 2 diabetes was a skyrocketing epidemic in America—up 40% between 1990 and 1999 alone. The reason? We're more and more overweight and less and less active.

An estimated 16 million Americans have diabetes, and at least one-third are undiagnosed and untreated. But lurking behind that troubling statistic is an even bigger, but barely mentioned, shadow epidemic: Some 20 to 30 million Americans probably have impaired glucose tolerance. Most don't know they have it. Those who do often dismiss it as "a touch of sugar" or "borderline diabetes." Their doctors may call it impaired glucose tolerance or impaired fasting glucose, depending on what test was used to diagnose it. But to underscore the danger that you shouldn't ignore, *Prevention* calls this invisible and often-dismissed condition early diabetes.

It's a health threat by any name, raising your risk of full-blown type 2 diabetes by 50% over 10 years and potentially doubling your risk of heart disease, tripling your risk of high blood pressure, and making you five times more likely to die from a heart attack. Researchers are also just beginning to suspect that there may be a link between high blood sugar and some forms of cancer.

But these dangers are often downplayed—if mentioned at all. "I refer to it as the Rodney Dangerfield of human diseases. It doesn't get any respect," says John Buse, MD, PhD, CDE (certified diabetes educator), associate professor of medicine at the University of North Carolina School of Medicine in Chapel Hill, and director of the university's Diabetes Care Center.

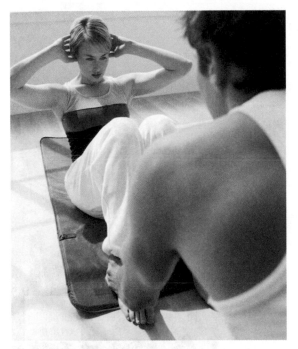

Keep impaired glucose tolerance from turning into full-blown diabetes by changing the way you eat and getting exercise.

Why Body Fat Matters

Genetics may account for 15 to 20% of diabetes and early diabetes risk. There's even new evidence that chronic lack of sleep can make you susceptible. But the real culprit is our high-fat, high-stress, no-time-for-exercise way of life and the epidemic of obesity that's come with it. Studies show that obesity raises diabetes risk by up to 93%. And inactivity alone raises the risk by 25%.

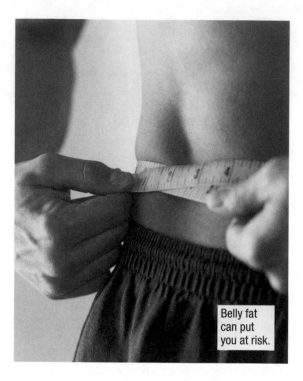

Belly fat can put you at risk.

Fifty-five percent of Americans are overweight, with a body mass index (BMI) of 25 or higher. (See "Know Your BMI" below.) And more than one-quarter have a BMI of 30 or higher, a level considered obese. More kids are overweight too. As a result, diabetes is on the rise and is becoming more common among younger people. The CDC estimates that the number of people in their 30s with type 2 diabetes has increased 70%. And among children, the disease has increased tenfold in the past 5 years.

TAKE CONTROL: Know Your BMI

To estimate body mass index, multiply your weight (in pounds) by 703. Multiply your height (in inches) by itself. Divide your first answer by your second answer.

Research also suggests that belly fat—or visceral fat, the kind that's packed around internal organs and is often linked to high levels of the stress hormone cortisol—may be an even more potent risk factor than weight alone. A study of 678 Hispanic and African-American people with a family history of diabetes found that regardless of age, gender, or weight, visceral fat was the most powerful factor in determining who had insulin resistance—the body's lack of sensitivity to insulin that causes early diabetes.

"Overweight, a high-fat diet, and visceral fat all intertwine to produce insulin resistance," says Dr. Buse. "We don't completely understand the process yet, but one theory is that people who are insulin-resistant are storing excess dietary fat in all kinds of inappropriate places, such as in muscle cells and in the liver, which makes it harder for their body to use sugar as fuel."

During early diabetes, scientists suspect that high insulin levels may raise heart disease risk into the danger zone by thickening artery walls and raising blood pressure. And insulin resistance is linked to the development of an extremely lethal kind of bad cholesterol—small, dense LDLs—that set the stage for heart disease.

The Simple Test You *Must* Have

Early diabetes is easy to detect with a simple blood check called a fasting plasma glucose test. After an 8- to 12-hour fast, your blood is drawn and blood sugar levels measured. A reading of 109 mg/dl or less is normal; 110 to 125 is called impaired fasting glucose—another name for impaired glucose tolerance; and 126 or higher is a sign of full-blown diabetes.

Prevention's "Stop Diabetes Before It Starts" Plan

Don't wait! Diabetes experts say these easy steps can dramatically reduce your risk of diabetes or reverse early diabetes.

1. Get tested now. See the risk factors and testing information in chapter 1.

2. And later. Get retested in 6 months to a year to find out if your risk has gone up or down.

3. Nudge the scale. Even extremely overweight people lowered their risk of diabetes by 70% when they lost just 5% of their body weight—even if they didn't exercise. If you weigh 175 lb, that's a little less than 9 lb.

4. Cut the fat. Targets for healthy fat intake range from less than 30% of daily calories (less than 10% saturated fat) to a daily 42 g fat. *Prevention* recommends keeping total fat intake to 25% of your daily calories.

5. Rev up the fruits, veggies, and whole grains. *Prevention* recommends nine servings of fruits and vegetables a day. Try to make at least half of your grain choices (including breads, rice, and pasta) whole grain to raise your fiber intake still higher.

6. Move a *little* more. People in a Finnish study who exercised the most—up to 4 hours a week—lowered their risk of diabetes by 80% even if they didn't lose any weight. America's Diabetes Prevention Program (DPP), which aims for just 30 minutes of exercise five times a week, also got big results. Moderate exercise—walking, biking, playing tennis—is enough to improve your odds.

7. Befriend your diary. In two different studies, keeping a food diary kept participants on track to eating better. List what you eat, the portion sizes, and fat content.

8. Enlist a coach. The secret to the success of study volunteers was attendance at regular meetings with a registered dietitian/lifestyle counselor. "She became like my shrink, helping me get through stressful times without overeating and figuring out how to help me get past obstacles to healthier habits," says DPP participant Maureen Marinelli.

Your insurance plan may not cover nutrition counseling if you're diagnosed with early diabetes. But it may if you have another health problem such as high cholesterol, high triglycerides, high blood pressure, or obesity. It's worth asking. Otherwise, try a program such as Weight Watchers, or log on to www.prevention.com and sign in at our message boards on weight loss and nutrition.

Ask your doctor to test you.

New evidence suggests that the oral glucose tolerance test may catch early diabetes sooner—and may also be a more accurate test for people over 65.

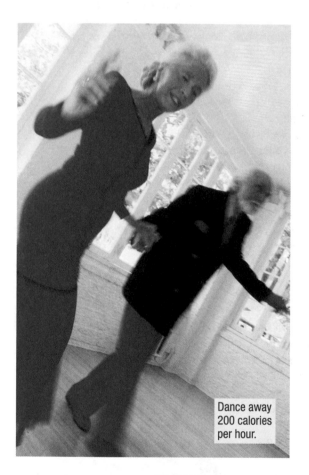

Dance away 200 calories per hour.

Another check, called the oral glucose tolerance test, involves drinking a sugared beverage and getting a blood sugar check after 2 hours. If your result is between 140 and 199 mg/dl, you have impaired glucose tolerance; 200 or higher indicates diabetes.

Which test is better? New evidence suggests that the oral glucose tolerance test may catch early diabetes sooner—and may also be a more accurate test for people over 65. Who should be tested? Probably everyone, but if you fit the high-risk profile for diabetes, get yourself tested as soon as possible.

"Knowing your blood sugar level is as important as knowing your cholesterol levels," says Robert Sherwin, MD, past president of the American Diabetes Association and director of the Diabetes Endocrinology Research Center at Yale University. "Some day, that will be common."

Cut Your Risk by 80%

You can lower your risk of getting full-blown diabetes by 80 to 100% by losing as little as 5% of your body weight—just 8 lb if you weigh 160, for example (multiply your weight times .05)—and exercising as little as half an hour a day. As a bonus, you'll also slash your heart disease risk.

That's what happened in the Finnish Diabetes Prevention Study, when 523 extremely overweight people with impaired glucose tolerance tried this easy-does-it, five-point plan:

1. Get half an hour of exercise daily.
2. Lose 5% of your total weight.
3. Reduce your fat intake to 30% of total calories.

30 Ways to Get Your 30 Minutes a Day

There are plenty of choices when it comes to picking an exercise. Just look down this list to get some ideas and to see how many calories you can expect to burn. No matter which activity you choose, your body will get the healthy workout it needs. Remember, you're shooting for 30 minutes of exercise five times a week. (Note: These figures are based on a 150-lb person. If you weigh more, you'll burn more calories. If you weigh less, you'll burn fewer.)

Exercise	Calories Burned
Aerobics classes and videotapes	228 per ½ hour
Bicycling	130–145 per ½ hour, depending on speed and terrain
Cross-country skiing	243–558 per ½ hour, depending on speed and terrain
Cross-country ski machine	254–339 per ½ hour, depending on intensity
Dancing, per ½ hour	
Ballroom	105
Modern	147
Country line	150
Aerobic	201–276
Elliptical training	250–300 per hour
Hiking	250 per ½ hour
Inline skating	170–238 per ½ hour, depending on speed and terrain
Jogging and treadmill running	102 per mile
Jumping rope	110–130 per 10 minutes
Power walking	198–250 per mile
Rowing machine	240–360 per ½ hour
Spinning	535 per 45-minute class
Stationary cycling	130–330 per ½ hour
Step aerobics	300 per ½ hour, using a 6" step
Stepping or stairclimbing machine	250–350 per ½ hour
Swimming	249–351 per ½ hour, depending on stroke and speed
Tennis	237 per ½ hour in a highly competitive match
Walking	100 per mile
Water aerobics	200–250 per ½ hour
Outdoor chores, per ½ hour	
Raking	111
Hoeing	186
Mowing	228
Digging	258

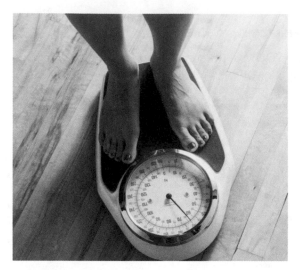

You can lower your risk of getting full-blown diabetes by 80 to 100% by losing as little as 5% of your body weight.

4. Cut your saturated fat intake to less than 10% of total calories.

5. Eat more fiber (fruits, veggies, and whole grains).

Those who took four of the five steps didn't develop diabetes at all. Those who lost the weight and reached two other goals reduced their risk by more than 70%. And those who said they exercised consistently and succeeded at reaching at least two other goals cut their risk by 80%.

"Of course we celebrated when we got the results," says lead investigator Jaakko Tuomilehto, MD, PhD, academy professor in the diabetes and genetic epidemiology unit of Finland's National Public Health Institute in Helsinki. "We think the biggest long-range health bene-

fits will probably be a reduction in the risk of cardiovascular and renal (kidney) complications and a reduction in the risk of all other major diabetes complications."

Americans should expect the same results, say US researchers, who recently released the findings of the landmark $174 million Diabetes Prevention Program (DPP)—a study that was ended a year early because the results were so dramatic. Among its 3,224 participants (all of whom had impaired glucose tolerance), those who lost 5 to 7% of their body weight and exercised for half an hour a day reduced their risk of developing full-blown type 2 diabetes by a whopping 58%. In contrast, those who took a diabetes drug (tested to see if it would reduce diabetes risk) improved their odds by only 31%. "Every year that a person can live free of diabetes means an added year of life free of suffering, disability, and the medical costs incurred by this disease," says Edward Horton, MD, professor of medicine at Harvard Medical School and director of clinical research at the Joslin Diabetes Center in Boston, where he is lead investigator for Joslin's part in the DPP.

You can take control of early diabetes right now by following the tips in *Prevention*'s "Stop Diabetes Before It Starts" Plan. Then check out our simple 10-step eating plan in chapter 5. It covers all the foods you need (including what to eat less of) to meet our diabetes prevention guidelines.

To meet our exercise recommendation of 30 minutes five times a week, start with "30 Ways to Get Your 30 Minutes a Day" on p. 27. And for even more exercise options, including a great walking plan that lowers blood sugar, take a look at "Exercise Prescriptions for Diabetes" in part 4 of this book.

CHAPTER 5

The Diabetes-Blocking Diet

Get all the nutrition you need to prevent diabetes— and lose weight at the same time

A healthy diet is at the heart of any diabetes prevention plan. Eating right helps keep blood sugar and fats at steady levels, which is the key to keeping diabetes at bay.

That where our Diabetes-Blocking Diet comes in. It takes care of all the diet recommendations found in *Prevention*'s "Stop Diabetes Before It Starts" Plan. It's rich in nutrient-dense fruits, vegetables, and whole grains, is low in fat, and it will also help you meet that goal of losing 5% of your total body weight. In addition, this exclusive diet offers protection against other health risks such as heart disease and cancer.

Just start following these 10 steps, and you'll be well on your way to taking control of your diabetes!

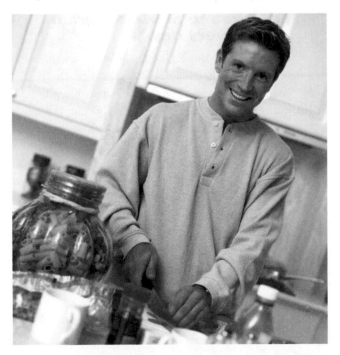

Step 1

Eat nine servings of fruit and vegetables every day.

Fruit and vegetables are the foundation of the Diabetes-Blocking Diet—as opposed to grains, the foundation of the traditional USDA Food Guide Pyramid. You'll be eating nine ½-cup servings of a variety of fruits and veggies a day. Sound like overkill? In reality, it could spell extra life. Study after study links diets highest in fruits and vegetables with less incidence of diabetes and many other diseases.

More and more experts are saying that five a day should be the minimum and that nine a day—five vegetables and four fruits—is the optimum. Yet most Americans get only four a day. In the Diabetes-Blocking Diet, you'll need to make every meal and snack a fruit or veggie opportunity.

Step 2

Eat three to six whole grain foods every day.

Diets high in whole grains are linked to less diabetes (and less heart disease, stroke, and cancer). If you've been eating a high-carbohydrate diet with lots of refined grains—typically breads, rolls, bagels, pretzels, and crackers made from white flour—it may be a challenge at first to find whole grain substitutes. But the payoff is worth it. To your body, refined white flour is the same as sugar, making a diet high in white flour foods the same as a high-sugar diet.

Whole grains also mean extra fiber, which is the closest thing to a magic bullet for weight loss. Not only does it fill you up quickly with fewer calories, but it also eliminates some of the calories

TAKE CONTROL: Save Time

Use timesaving frozen and canned veggies and fruits, which provide as much nutrition as fresh produce.

you eat! Fiber whisks calories through your digestive system so quickly that some of them never have a chance to end up on your hips.

To maximize fiber's slimming powers, aim for 25 to 35 g daily. By eating 30 g a day, your body will absorb almost 120 fewer calories a day. That adds up to a 13-lb weight loss in 1 year!

Step 3

Eat two or three calcium-rich foods every day.

This is great advice for everyone, not just for people with early diabetes. Adequate calcium not only supports strong bones and helps prevent osteoporosis, but clinical studies suggest that it also helps prevent colon cancer, high blood pressure, and PMS. And calcium may lower your body fat. A group of women who ate at least 1,000 mg calcium a day as part of a diet of no more than 1,900 daily calories lost more weight—as much as 6 lb more—during a 2-year study than women who ate less calcium.

Obvious high-calcium choices include 1% and fat-free milk, low-fat and fat-free yogurt, and reduced-fat and fat-free cheese. Other good choices are orange and grapefruit juices and soy milk that have been fortified with calcium; to equal the calcium found in milk, look for at least 30% of the Daily Value (DV) for calcium per serving.

If you're 50 or older or have low bone density, you should be getting 1,500 mg calcium a day. If you're younger, aim for 1,000 mg a day.

Step 4

Eat beans at least five times a week.

Beans are the highest-fiber foods you can find, with the single exception of breakfast cereals made with wheat bran. Diets high in fiber are linked to less diabetes and other chronic diseases such as cancer, heart disease, stroke, and even ulcers. Beans are especially high in soluble fiber, which lowers cholesterol levels, and folate, which lowers levels of another risk factor for heart disease: homocysteine.

Step 5

Snack on nuts five times a week.

People with diabetes are at increased risk of heart disease. And studies show that people who eat nuts regularly have less heart disease and other illness than people who avoid them. Even among the healthiest eaters, the ones who also eat nuts

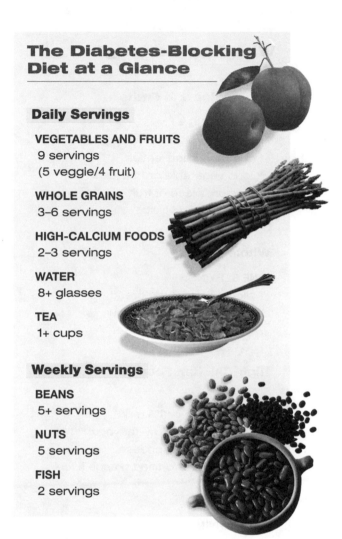

The Diabetes-Blocking Diet at a Glance

Daily Servings

VEGETABLES AND FRUITS
9 servings
(5 veggie/4 fruit)

WHOLE GRAINS
3–6 servings

HIGH-CALCIUM FOODS
2–3 servings

WATER
8+ glasses

TEA
1+ cups

Weekly Servings

BEANS
5+ servings

NUTS
5 servings

FISH
2 servings

have the best health records. Exactly why isn't known yet, but one reason could be compounds in nuts called tocotrienols.

The key to eating nuts is moderation; they're so high in calories that you could easily gain weight. To avoid temptation, keep a jar of chopped nuts in your fridge. Sprinkle 2 tablespoons a day on cereal, yogurt, veggies, salads, or wherever the crunch and rich flavor appeal to you.

What's a Serving?

Vegetables and Fruits

ONE SERVING =
½ cup cooked or raw veggie
1 cup raw green leaves
¾ cup vegetable or fruit juice
1 medium piece of fruit
½ cup chopped fruit

Whole Grains

ONE SERVING =
1 slice whole wheat bread
½ cup brown rice or bulgur
½ cup whole wheat pasta

High-Calcium Foods

ONE SERVING =
1 cup fat-free or 1% milk
1 cup fat-free or low-fat yogurt
1 oz reduced-fat cheese
1 cup calcium-fortified orange juice

Beans

ONE SERVING =
½ cup cooked dried beans/lentils

Nuts

ONE SERVING = 2 tablespoons, chopped

Fish

ONE SERVING = 3 oz cooked

Step 6

Eat fish twice a week.

Fish is another heart protector; studies show that people who eat fish twice a week have fewer fatal heart attacks. Scientists credit omega-3 fats, which have the ability to prevent the development of a dangerously irregular heartbeat.

The protein in fish is also a great hunger stopper—and it helps build healthy muscles that burn tons of calories. "Fish is an excellent source of protein, because it's high in omega-3 fatty acids that are good for your heart while being low in cholesterol and saturated fat," says Michael Hamilton, MD, MPH, former program and medical director of the Diet and Fitness Center at Duke University in Durham, NC. "And protein is important for promoting satiety, the feeling of fullness you look for in a meal." To get the most omega-3s, choose salmon, white albacore tuna canned in water, rainbow trout, anchovies, herring, sardines, and mackerel.

Step 7

Drink eight glasses of water every day, plus a cup or more of tea.

Every cell in your body needs water to function. Not only does drinking lots of water help you feel full (and eat less), but big water drinkers also appear to get less colon and bladder cancer. Every cup of tea you drink provides a strong infusion of antioxidants that help keep blood from clotting too easily (which may thwart heart attacks—important to people with early diabetes). Antioxidants may also help lower your risk of cancer and rheumatoid arthritis.

Step 8

Follow a fat budget.

To stay within a healthy fat budget—25% of calories from fat—you must find the maximum fat allowance for your calorie level (see chart below).

Once you know your fat budget, see whether you're staying within the bounds by adding up the grams of fat for all the food that you eat in a day. Try to get most of your fat from olive and canola oils (or salad dressings made from them), trans-free margarine, nuts, and fish. And spread your fat throughout the day—a little fat helps you absorb fat-soluble nutrients from vegetables and fruit.

Maximum Fat Allowance

Calories	Grams of Fat
1,250	35
1,500	42
1,750	49
2,000	56
2,250	63

Step 9

Take your vitamins.

In addition to your smart diet, take a moderate multivitamin/mineral supplement as a nutritional backup. You'll also want to add the following individual supplements, all of which are beneficial to blood sugar.

100 to 500 mg vitamin C. In one study, Italian researchers gave 40 people with diabetes

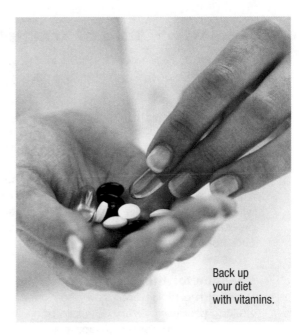

Back up your diet with vitamins.

1 g vitamin C every day. After 4 months, the patients' ability to use insulin had significantly improved, perhaps because vitamin C helps insulin penetrate cells.

100 to 400 IU vitamin E. When Finnish scientists studied 944 men, they found that those with the lowest levels of vitamin E in their blood were four times more likely to have diabetes than those with the highest levels. Vitamin E may somehow help insulin carry sugar from the blood into cells in muscles and tissues, the researchers speculate.

500 to 1,000 mg calcium. Whether you have early diabetes or not, you may not be getting enough of this mineral in your diet. On days when you eat only two calcium-rich foods, take 500 mg calcium (if you're under 50) or 1,000 mg calcium divided into two separate doses of 500 mg each (if you're 50 or older).

One Man's Tale of Triumph

Richard K. Daly learned firsthand just how powerfully a healthy diet and exercise can control high blood sugar. Here's his story.

The Wake-Up Call

"Over the years I back-and-forthed my weight up to 244 lb. I was tired most of the time, and I had an almost unquenchable thirst. The next thing I knew I was in the hospital, diagnosed with diabetes. I was there for 5 days, getting insulin to bring down my sky-high blood sugar and learning how to give myself insulin shots. However, it was the diabetes education classes, which drove home the importance of a healthy diet, exercise, checking product labels, and testing my blood sugar levels, that inspired me to take control.

Changes for the Better

"My first morning home from the hospital, I started a real walking program. Every day, rain or snow, I walked at least 35 minutes. My hospitalization also convinced me to start eating right. I began reading labels and buying unrefined foods such as fruits, vegetables, whole grain breads, and cereals instead of highly refined cakes and cookies. I also started eating oatmeal and bran cereal—with fat-free milk and raspberries or blueberries for more flavor. I'd eat three meals a day. About 2 or 3 hours after a meal, I'd have a snack—fruit, cottage cheese, a bagel, or carrots instead of chips. If I got an urge for something sweet, I'd have a piece of fruit instead of the usual Twinkie.

Living the Good Life

"A month after I got home from the hospital, I was off insulin and on just a small dose of medication. Within 2 months, I was off all drugs. My body fat started coming off even faster. A year after I left the hospital, my weight was down to 170 lb—a 74-lb loss! I've maintained it ever since. My waist is 10 inches smaller, and I'm fit, lean, and muscular. My blood sugar is below 100 [milligrams per deciliter of blood], from a high in the hospital of 290. My doctor still shakes his head in amazement at what I've accomplished. At 61, I feel better than ever!"

Trace Minerals That Make a Difference

Two minerals have been shown to stabilize blood sugar levels and to help guard against diabetic retinopathy, a serious eye complication.

Chromium. The trace mineral chromium improves the body's ability to regulate blood sugar. A cup of broccoli contains 22 micrograms (mcg), 18% of the Daily Value (DV). A 2½-oz waffle has almost 7 mcg, 6% of the DV, while a 3-oz serving of turkey ham has 10 mcg, 8% of the DV.

Magnesium. Experts estimate that 25% of people with diabetes are low in this mineral. And studies have shown that people with lower levels of magnesium in their diets or in their blood are more likely to develop type 2 diabetes. A good source of magnesium is baked halibut, which contains 91 mg magnesium per 3-oz serving, 23% of the DV. And a ½-cup serving of long grain brown rice has 42 mg, 11% of the DV.

Step 10

Give indulgences careful consideration.

These choices are up to you with the Diabetes-Blocking Diet.

Meat and poultry. If you want, you can have up to 3 cooked oz a day (the size of a deck of cards). You'll get enough protein in this diet without adding meat, and studies consistently link vegetarian diets to better health, perhaps partly because diets low in meat are naturally lower in saturated fat.

Eggs. If you have diabetes or high cholesterol or are overweight, you can safely eat up to four eggs a week; otherwise, up to seven eggs a week is permissible.

Alcohol. Whether you can drink alcohol with diabetes largely depends on the medication that you're taking. See "Forbidden Foods You Can Order" on p. 59 for more on this subject.

Sweets. Reserve these for special occasions. Talk to your doctor or a registered dietitian if you'd like to work sweets into your diet. In general, it's a good idea to avoid high-sugar foods, which offer lots of empty calories and not much else.

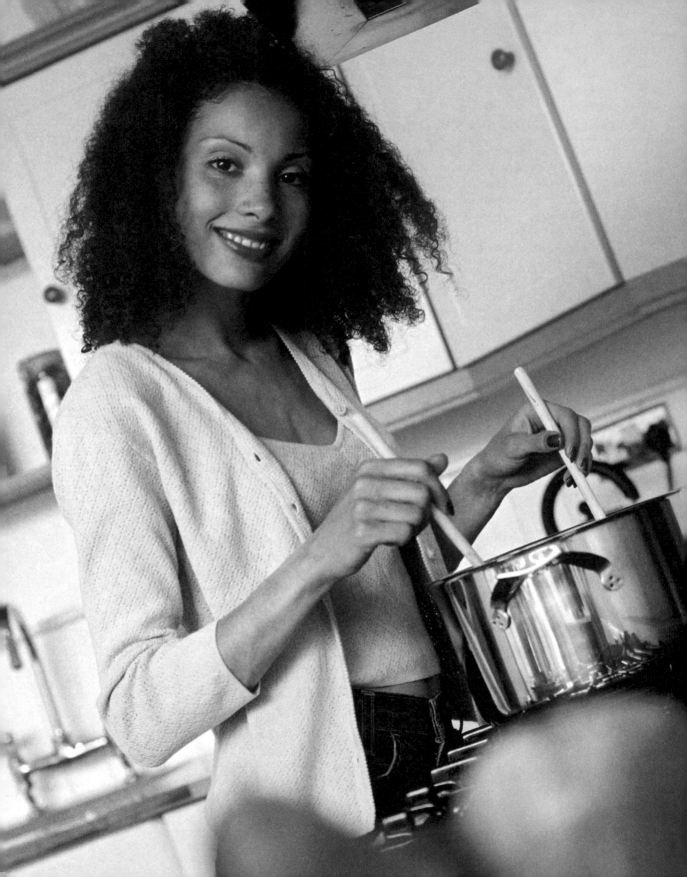

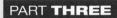

PART THREE

Eat to Beat Diabetes

Take control of this disease by simply choosing more of the right foods

CHAPTER 6

The Diabetes Food Exchange System

Follow this plan, and you'll get all the nutrition you need for optimal diabetes control

You already know that eating well is an essential part of managing diabetes. The right foods can help to keep your blood sugar and fats at steady levels—and that's key to both taking control of diabetes and avoiding diabetes-related problems. Studies show that people with type 2 diabetes who ate a high-fiber, high–complex carbohydrate diet improved their blood sugar control by an average of 95%! And those with type 1 diabetes experienced a considerable 30% improvement.

The Diabetes Food Exchange System is an easy way to make sure you're getting the right amounts of fiber-rich, low-fat foods and other wholesome, healing nutrients. Just read up on how to use it, and then put the exchange system to work for you!

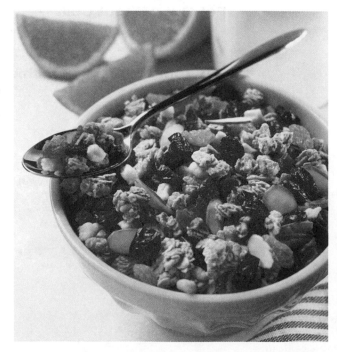

Diabetes Exchanges Explained

The exchange system is a food grouping program organized by the American Dietetic Association and the American Diabetes Association (ADA). This system has a greater level of detail than the diabetes food pyramid (see p. 43), and it's easy to keep track of what you eat—whether you're trying to control your diabetes, lose weight, or both.

To use the exchange system, determine your target calorie level based on whether you need to maintain your weight or lose weight. (See "How Many Calories Do You Need?" at right.) We recommend losing 1 to 2 lb a week for optimal weight loss. Then see "Find Your Exchange Allowance" on p. 40 to see how many servings of the various food groups you should eat each day. All the recipes in this book (starting on p. 105) include dietary exchanges to simplify meal planning.

But first, read "How Much Is an Exchange Serving?" below to learn just how big an exchange serving is.

How Much Is an Exchange Serving?

Knowing serving sizes is crucial to making any meal plan work. Unfortunately, because more of us are eating in restaurants (where the portions are

How Many Calories Do You Need?

Here's a way to quickly estimate how many calories you should be eating. Just find your activity level in the chart below, then multiply that number by your weight in pounds. Use the resulting "calorie needs" number to look up your exchange allowance on p. 40.

1. Find Your Activity Level

If you are a . . .	Your activity level is . . .
Sedentary woman	12
Sedentary man	13
Lightly active woman	14
Lightly active man	15
Active woman	16
Active man	17
Very active woman	18
Very active man	20

2. Determine Your Calorie Needs

Note: If you're trying to lose weight, use your goal weight instead of your actual weight.
   Activity Level x Weight in Pounds = Calorie Needs

Studies show that those with type 2 diabetes who ate a high-fiber, high–complex carbohydrate diet improved their blood sugar control by an average of 95%!

Find Your Exchange Allowance

In the chart below, pick the "calorie needs" level that is closest to the one you (preferably with the help of a dietitian) have chosen to maintain your current weight or to reach your goal weight. Then scan the food groups to see how many servings of each food to eat in a day. These numbers are meant only as a guide. Some days you may end up eating more or less in any given food category.

Food Group	Daily Calorie Needs				
	1,200	1,500	1,800	2,000	2,500
Bread	5	6	8	9	10
Fruit	3	3	5	5	6
Milk	1½	2	2	2	4
Vegetable	2	5	5	5	5
Meat	5	6	6	8	10
Fat	3	4	5	5	6

huge), we've gotten accustomed to eating more than we should. The average take-out muffin is about five times the size it should be. Even healthy foods such as potatoes are nearly three times the size that health experts recommend. When in doubt as to what makes a serving, minimize—don't supersize. Here are the specifics of exchange servings. (Some of these vary from food pyramid serving sizes. See "The Diabetes Food Pyramid" on p. 43 for a comparison.)

Bread. Sometimes called starches, the bread group encompasses all carbohydrate-rich foods, such as cereals, grains, pastas, breads, crackers, and

Knowing serving sizes is crucial to making any meal plan work.

snacks. Starchy vegetables such as corn, green peas, plantains, potatoes, winter squash, and yams are also included here. In general, one serving (cooked, where applicable) is . . .

- ½ cup cereal, grain, pasta, or starchy vegetable
- 1 slice bread
- 1 oz of most snack foods (See "Treats" on p. 42 for a detailed list.)

Fruit. These can be fresh, frozen, canned, or dried fruit or fruit juice. One fruit serving equals . . .

- 1 small to medium piece of fresh fruit
- ½ cup canned fruit (with a small amount of juice), cut fruit, or fruit juice
- ¼ cup dried fruit

Milk. Fat-free milk and yogurt are included here. To count cheeses, see the meat group. Cream and other dairy fats are counted in the fat group. One serving of milk equals . . .

- 1 cup (½ pint or 8 fluid oz) fat-free milk
- 1 cup fat-free or low-fat yogurt

Vegetable. This includes all vegetables except the starchy ones mentioned above. Go for the richest colors you can find. Dark green and dark yellow vegetables are the most nutritious. These include spinach, broccoli, romaine lettuce, carrots, bell peppers, and chile peppers. In general, one vegetable serving is . . .

- ½ cup cooked vegetables or vegetable juice
- 1 cup raw vegetables

Meat. When buying meats, choose those

> **TAKE CONTROL:** Shop Wisely
>
> Use our shopping list on p. 178 the next time you head to the supermarket. This list will help ensure that you have all sorts of healthy foods on hand, and it will make it easier for you to stick to a well-balanced diet.

labeled "lean" or "very lean." "Select" and "choice" grades are leaner than "prime." Look for ground beef rather than meat labeled "hamburger," because the latter may contain more fat. In addition to meats, this group includes other protein-based foods such as cheese, eggs, and beans.

Meal Planning Principles

Try to follow these basic eating guidelines recommended by the American Diabetes Association to help keep your blood sugar in balance.

Establish consistent eating patterns. Don't skip meals, whether you're on diabetes medication or not. Skipping meals can lead to low blood sugar levels, and overeating to make up for a missed meal can lead to high blood sugar.

Eat a variety of foods. This will ensure you get proper nutrition. The easiest way to get a variety of foods is to follow the exchange program or the diabetes food pyramid.

Control carbohydrates. Aim for 45 to 75 g carbohydrates per meal and no more than 15 to 30 g per snack. Both refined sugars (such as sweets) and naturally occurring carbs (such as from grains, fruits, vegetables, and milk) count.

Eat less fat. People with diabetes have a higher risk of heart disease, so it's best to follow a low-fat diet.

Eat more fiber. Most of us don't get enough fiber. The recommended daily intake is 25 to 35 g. You can get fiber from whole grain breads, cereals, whole fruit, vegetables, and dried beans and peas.

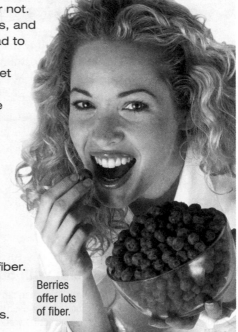

Berries offer lots of fiber.

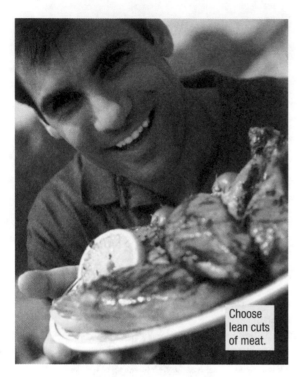

Choose lean cuts of meat.

- 1 oz cooked lean beef, pork, lamb, skinless poultry, fish, or shellfish
- 1 oz cheese
- ½ cup cooked dried beans, peas, or lentils
- 1 egg

Fat. Most fats have the same number of calories per serving. But some fats are better for you than others. The good monounsaturated and polyunsaturated fats are generally found in plant foods such as olive oil and nuts and in some seafood. Generally, one serving of fat equals . . .

- 1 teaspoon butter, regular margarine, or vegetable oil
- 1 tablespoon regular salad dressing
- ⅛ of one medium avocado
- 8 to 10 olives
- 6 to 10 nuts
- 2 teaspoons peanut butter
- 2 teaspoons tahini paste
- 1 tablespoon sesame seeds
- 1 slice bacon
- 2 tablespoons half-and-half
- 2 tablespoons coconut
- 3 tablespoons reduced-fat sour cream

Bacon is counted in the fat group. Note that the serving size for meat and cheese is 1 oz. But don't worry, you can still eat plenty of meat. We recommend that you get somewhere between 5 and 10 servings (5 to 10 oz) from the meat group each day. (You'll find your recommended number of servings in "Find Your Exchange Allowance" on p. 40.) Just remember that there may be several ounces (or several servings) of meat in any one meal you eat. Generally, one serving of meat equals . . .

Treats. You've probably gotten used to many of the foods that you consider treats. If a little bit helps you stick to a healthy eating plan, there's no reason to stop eating these foods. Just eat moderate amounts, and make sure you keep track of them. Here's how to count treats using the exchange system. Note that things such as sherbet and jelly are included in the bread

TAKE CONTROL: Be Careful with Sugar

Sugar is allowed, but indulge with care. The American Diabetes Association (ADA) changed its rules in 1994, making sugar an okay-in-strict-moderation food. Sugar counts as a carbohydrate and must be substituted for other foods containing carbohydrates. The ADA recommends working with your dietitian to set up a meal plan.

The Diabetes Food Pyramid

The American Diabetes Association's diabetes food pyramid is a variation of the USDA Food Guide Pyramid that you're probably already familiar with. If you choose to use the diabetes food pyramid as a guide, take note that a few of its servings are different in size than a diabetes exchange serving. The differences are listed below.

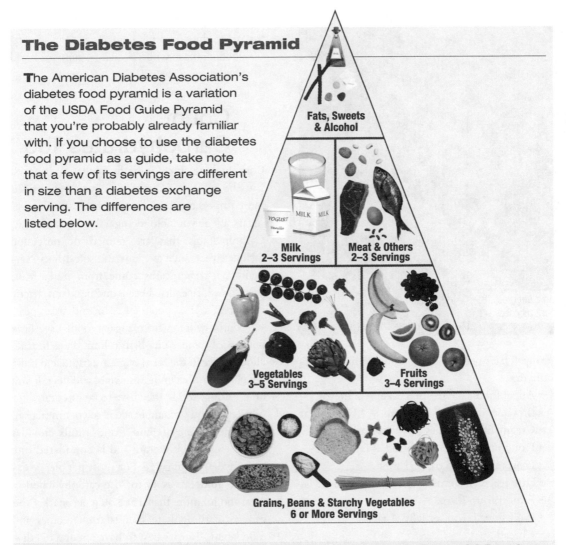

Fats, Sweets & Alcohol

Milk
2–3 Servings

Meat & Others
2–3 Servings

Vegetables
3–5 Servings

Fruits
3–4 Servings

Grains, Beans & Starchy Vegetables
6 or More Servings

Food	Diabetes Exchange Serving	Diabetes Pyramid Serving
Lean meat, poultry, or fish	1 oz	2–3 oz
Cheese	1 oz (a meat exchange)	1½ oz
Dry cereal	½ cup (a bread exchange)	1 oz
Fruit juice	½ cup	¾ cup
Peanut butter	2 teaspoons (a fat exchange)	2 tablespoons (a meat group serving)

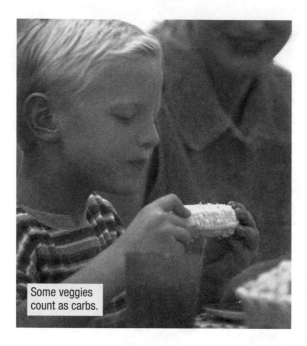

Some veggies count as carbs.

• Potato chips or tortilla chips (1 oz) = 1 bread, 2 fat
• Pudding made with 1% milk (½ cup) = 2 bread
• Sherbet or sorbet (½ cup) = 2 bread

Count Carbohydrates Too

Carbohydrates include both starches and sugars. But the total amount of carbs you consume is more important than the type; both starches and sugars affect your blood sugar in the same way. Carbohydrates that are refined or processed include sweets such as candy and soft drinks. Naturally occurring carbs come from milk, fruit, pasta, bread, rice, dried beans and peas, and starchy vegetables such as potatoes, corn, and green peas.

Carbohydrates from sugary foods have little nutritional value, so it's best to limit these. Instead, choose carbs in the form of grains, fruits, and milk, which contain vitamins, minerals, and fiber. If you do eat sugary foods, they have to be substituted for other carbs and not simply added to your meal plan.

One serving of grain, fruit, or milk provides about 15 g carbohydrate and is considered one carbohydrate exchange. For most people, a reasonable guideline is 45 to 75 g carbohydrate per meal and no more than 15 to 30 g per snack. (You can get carbohydrate counts from recipes and food labels.) But it's best to have a registered dietitian develop a meal plan that meets your individual requirements.

group. That's because these foods are mostly carbohydrates.

• Angel food cake (¹⁄₁₂ of a cake) = 2 bread
• Brownie, unfrosted (2" square) = 1 bread, 1 fat
• Cream-filled cookies (2) = 1 bread, 1 fat
• Doughnut, plain = 1½ bread, 2 fat
• Fruit juice bar (3 oz) = 1 fruit
• Fruit pie, with 2 crusts (⅙ of pie) = 3 bread, 2 fat
• Fruit roll-up (¾ oz) = 1 fruit
• Fruit spread, jam, or jelly (1 tablespoon) = 1 bread
• Hot dog (1 oz) = 1 meat
• Ice cream (½ cup) = 1 bread, 2 fat

TAKE CONTROL: Avoid the Trans Fats

A recent study showed that high intakes of trans fatty acids may increase your risk of developing type 2 diabetes. Trans fatty acids are found in margarine and foods cooked in hydrogenated vegetable oil, such as crackers, potato chips, cookies, and cakes. Reduce your risk by cutting back on stick margarine, using canola or olive oil for cooking, and limiting the aforementioned foods.

CHAPTER 7

Take Advantage of the Glycemic Index

Learn how to pick good carbs over bad ones to help balance your blood sugar

The glycemic index (or GI for short), which ranks carbohydrate foods by their effect on your blood sugar levels, was invented in the early 1980s by University of Toronto researchers as a tool to help control diabetes. Today it's an accepted diet strategy for helping control diabetes in Canada, Australia, England, and elsewhere.

Low-GI foods are the ones on which people with diabetes need to base their diets, and the glycemic index helps you identify and choose those good-for-you carbs over the less healthy, high-GI options. With our easy guide to more than 100 popular foods on p. 48, you can use the glycemic index to pick meals and snacks that give you an edge against diabetes—and may help you lose weight as well.

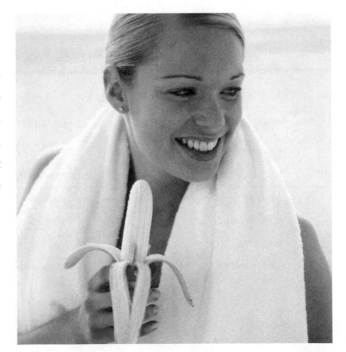

Carbs and Your Blood Sugar

The glycemic index assigns carbohydrate-containing foods a number based on how they affect your blood sugar, or blood glucose, after you eat them. Foods with a GI less than 55 cause only a little blip in blood sugar; those in the 55 to 70 range raise it a little higher; and carbs with GIs greater than 70 send blood sugar soaring. We're learning that low-GI carbs are healthy; high-GI carbs, in excess, are not.

What explains the difference in numbers? No matter what form the carb initially takes—the lactose in milk, the starch in a bagel, the sucrose in table sugar—your body eventually breaks it down to glucose. Glucose winds up in your bloodstream, fueling your cells. What makes a GI number high or low is how quickly the food breaks down during digestion. The longer your body has to wrestle with the carb to break it down into glucose, the slower the rise in blood glucose and the lower the GI.

Whole wheat bread won't cause the same spike in your blood sugar as French bread.

But it's not always easy to predict a food's GI. Fiber-rich foods often have lower GIs. Fiber, especially the soluble type in oats and beans, creates a web in the intestines that traps carb particles. Not surprisingly, beans have low GI numbers.

But when fiber is ground finely as it often is in whole wheat flour, it doesn't present enough of a digestive challenge to lower the GI of these foods. That explains why whole wheat bread has a GI number nearly identical to white bread. (But whole wheat bread is still a healthier choice than white, because of its extra fiber and other nutrients.)

Surprisingly, table sugar has a lower GI than potatoes. That's because it's made of two sugars, glucose and fructose; the glucose sails right into the bloodstream, but the fructose has to detour

Easy Low-GI Substitutes

Here are a few quick and easy ways to sneak low-GI foods into your regular diet.

High-GI Favorite	Lower-GI Choice
French bread, 95	100% stone-ground whole wheat bread, 53
Jelly beans, 80	Dried apricots, 31
Mashed or baked potato, 73 or 85	Roasted sweet potato, 54
Pretzels, 83	Popcorn, 55
Side of bread stuffing mix, 74	Side of canned baked beans, 48
Vanilla wafers, 77	Oatmeal cookies, 55

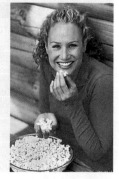

Six Secrets to Make the Glycemic Index Work for You

1. Eat one per meal. Try to choose one-third to one-half of your daily starches from the low-GI list. You're well on your way if you include one low-GI starch—for instance, a bowl of old-fashioned oatmeal, ½ cup beans, or some lentil soup—per meal.

2. Go whole grain. There are exceptions, but in general whole grain–based foods such as barley and bulgur have a low GI, mainly because their high fiber content slows digestion.

3. Rough it up. The less processed and rougher the grain or flour, the lower the GI. That's why pasta, which is made from a coarse-milled wheat, has a low GI even if it's not whole grain.

4. Bring it down low. Only have time to make instant rice? Just add some beans. Throwing in a low-GI food brings down the GI rating of the entire meal. Adding some fat or protein also lowers the GI level.

5. Be savvy about snacks. When you snack, you tend to have just one food, all by itself. That's fine if you're having a low-cal snack, whether the GI is high or not. But if you're having a high-GI bagel or doughnut with hundreds of calories, the glucose won't get blunted by other foods. So avoid starchy, high-GI foods as snacks.

6. Load up on fruits, vegetables, and legumes. Most have a low GI, and you'd have to eat pounds of the ones that don't to affect blood sugar. But by the same token, don't binge on low-GI foods that are high in calories, such as Snickers bars. Gaining weight will raise your blood sugar too.

through the liver, where it slowly gets converted into glucose. But the starch molecules in potatoes are strings of glucose. Boiling, baking, or mashing a potato causes the starch molecules to burst, making it easy for glucose to enter the bloodstream.

Benefits for Those with Diabetes

The good news is that sticking to a low-GI diet results in a minimum outpouring of insulin, and that has healthy ramifications all over your body. Here's what a low-GI diet appears to help you do.

Outsmart diabetes. "The beauty of the glycemic index for diabetics is that it not only helps control blood sugar and insulin, but its appetite-suppressing effects help them lose weight. And weight loss alone can reverse type 2 diabetes," declares Marc Rendell, MD, director of the Creighton Diabetes Center at Creighton University in Omaha, NE, and medical director of the Rose Salter Medical Research Foundation in Baltimore. Although he believes it's entirely possible to induce remission of many cases of type 2 diabetes using the glycemic index, he urges patients with diabetes to continue their current therapies and only add low-GI foods in consultation with a physician or registered dietitian.

continued on p. 50

The Glycemic Index of Popular Foods

LOW-GLYCEMIC INDEX FOODS
Less than 55

*Eat sparingly low-GI foods marked with an asterisk; these are high in empty calories.

Low-fat yogurt, artificially sweetened	14
Peanuts	14
Fructose	23
Plum	24
Grapefruit	25
Pearled barley	25
Peach	28
Canned peaches, natural juice	30
Dried apricots	31
Soy milk	31
Baby lima beans, frozen	32
Fat-free milk	32
Fettuccine	32
Low-fat yogurt, sugar sweetened	33
* M&M's Chocolate Candies, Peanut	33
Apple	36
Pear	36
Whole wheat spaghetti	37
Tomato soup	38
Apple juice	41
* Snickers bar	41
Spaghetti	41
All-Bran	42
Canned chickpeas	42
Custard	43
Grapes	43
Orange	43
Canned lentil soup	44
Canned pinto beans	45
Macaroni	45
Pineapple juice	46

Banana bread	47
Long grain rice	47
Parboiled rice	47
Bulgur	48
Canned baked beans	48
Grapefruit juice	48
Green peas	48
* Chocolate bar	49
Old-fashioned oatmeal	49
Cheese tortellini	50
* Low-fat ice cream	50
Canned kidney beans	52
Kiwifruit	52
Banana	53
100% stone-ground whole wheat bread	53
* Potato chips	54
* Pound cake	54
Special K	54
Sweet potato	54

INTERMEDIATE-GLYCEMIC INDEX FOODS
55 to 70

* Eat sparingly intermediate-GI foods marked with an asterisk; these are high in empty calories.

Brown rice	55
Canned fruit cocktail	55
Linguine	55
Oatmeal cookies	55
Popcorn	55
Sweet corn	55
White rice	56
Orange juice from frozen concentrate	57
Pita	57
Canned peaches, heavy syrup	58
Mini shredded wheats	58
Multi-Bran Chex	58

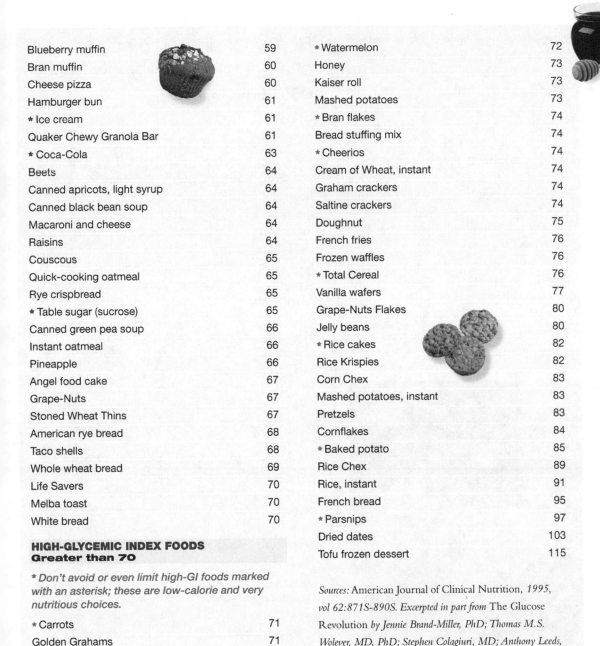

Blueberry muffin	59
Bran muffin	60
Cheese pizza	60
Hamburger bun	61
* Ice cream	61
Quaker Chewy Granola Bar	61
* Coca-Cola	63
Beets	64
Canned apricots, light syrup	64
Canned black bean soup	64
Macaroni and cheese	64
Raisins	64
Couscous	65
Quick-cooking oatmeal	65
Rye crispbread	65
* Table sugar (sucrose)	65
Canned green pea soup	66
Instant oatmeal	66
Pineapple	66
Angel food cake	67
Grape-Nuts	67
Stoned Wheat Thins	67
American rye bread	68
Taco shells	68
Whole wheat bread	69
Life Savers	70
Melba toast	70
White bread	70

HIGH-GLYCEMIC INDEX FOODS
Greater than 70

* Don't avoid or even limit high-GI foods marked with an asterisk; these are low-calorie and very nutritious choices.

* Carrots	71
Golden Grahams	71
Bagel	72
Corn chips	72

* Watermelon	72
Honey	73
Kaiser roll	73
Mashed potatoes	73
* Bran flakes	74
Bread stuffing mix	74
* Cheerios	74
Cream of Wheat, instant	74
Graham crackers	74
Saltine crackers	74
Doughnut	75
French fries	76
Frozen waffles	76
* Total Cereal	76
Vanilla wafers	77
Grape-Nuts Flakes	80
Jelly beans	80
* Rice cakes	82
Rice Krispies	82
Corn Chex	83
Mashed potatoes, instant	83
Pretzels	83
Cornflakes	84
* Baked potato	85
Rice Chex	89
Rice, instant	91
French bread	95
* Parsnips	97
Dried dates	103
Tofu frozen dessert	115

Sources: American Journal of Clinical Nutrition, *1995, vol 62:871S-890S. Excerpted in part from* The Glucose Revolution *by Jennie Brand-Miller, PhD; Thomas M.S. Wolever, MD, PhD; Stephen Colagiuri, MD; Anthony Leeds, MD; and Kaye Foster-Powell, M. Nutr. & Diet.*

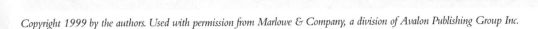

So far, research testing low- versus high-GI diets for diabetics is promising. A 1999 Swedish study of type 2 diabetics found that 4 weeks on a low-GI diet lowered blood glucose and insulin by 30% compared with a high-GI diet. In a recent 4-month study led by the University of Toronto's Thomas Wolever, MD, PhD, a low-GI diet markedly improved insulin sensitivity in a group of prediabetic insulin-resistant people. "If these trends were sustained—and I'm trying to get money to extend the study—these people could probably avoid diabetes," predicts Dr. Wolever.

Which is exactly the implication of several large-scale diet surveys. In a 6-year study of male health professionals, those eating the lowest-GI diets were 25% less likely to get diabetes. In the landmark Nurses' Health Study, the most powerful diabetes protection—a drop in risk of one-

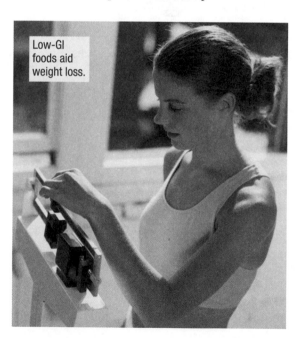

Low-GI foods aid weight loss.

Ready for dessert? Instead of a doughnut, enjoy lower-GI oatmeal cookies.

third or more—came from eating a low-GI diet and getting lots of fiber from cereal (7.5 g daily).

Drop pounds. Ever feel hungry just an hour or two after a meal? It could be because the meal had a high GI. Ironically, high-GI meals cause such a flood of insulin to cope with all the glucose that blood sugar levels wind up lower than if you'd never eaten. And low blood sugar may send out hunger alarms, according to Susan Roberts, PhD, professor of nutrition at Tufts University in Boston and author of *Feeding Your Child for Lifelong Health*. In one study, overweight children (average age 10) at Children's Hospital in Boston spent 4 months on either a low-GI diet or a low-fat diet of equal calories. The clear winner: the low-GI diet, with an average weight loss of 4.5 lb compared with 2.8 lb on the low-fat diet.

Dr. Roberts suspects that high-GI carbs are partly behind America's epidemic of obesity. "GI is not the complete answer to everyone's weight problem," she says. "But aside from the research, I am personally convinced that low-GI diets help people lose weight, myself included. My husband and I were eating a relatively high-GI instant oatmeal or low-GI Irish oatmeal for breakfast, and I'd call and ask how he felt 2 hours later. Both of us noticed a big decrease in hunger with the low-GI oatmeal. Now I've become very aware of the GI of what I eat and quite consistently find myself hungrier after very high-GI foods such as bagels, mashed potatoes, and the like." Of course, drop-

The Healing Power of Fiber

Fiber helps control glucose.

Many low-glycemic index foods are high in fiber, and research shows that increasing your fiber intake could help you avoid or delay the need for drugs to control your diabetes.

The research: In one study, 13 people with diabetes first ate a moderate-fiber diet, getting 8 g soluble fiber and 16 g insoluble fiber daily from produce, beans, and whole grains. After 6 weeks, they supercharged their fiber intake, raising it to 25 g each soluble and insoluble fiber, for a total fiber intake of 50 g. Researchers found that blood sugar levels were 10% lower on the 50-g-fiber eating plan. "That's comparable to what might occur with some medications for diabetes," says study author Abhimanyu Garg, MD, professor of internal medicine at the University of Texas Southwestern Medical Center in Dallas.

How it works: While we need both soluble and insoluble fiber each day, researchers suspect that soluble fiber may play an especially important role in glucose control, because it forms a thick gel that may interfere with carbohydrate and glucose absorption in the intestine. Soluble fiber also delays the movement of food into the small intestine, which slows postmeal surges in blood sugar, says Aaron Vinik, MD, PhD, director of the Strelitz Diabetes Research Institute in Norfolk, VA. The result: lower insulin levels and more manageable diabetes.

(Note: If your blood sugar is higher than 240 mg/dl, boosting your fiber intake probably won't eliminate the need for drugs, but a high-fiber diet can still improve your overall health.)

ping a few pounds is very beneficial to controlling your blood sugar too.

Keep your heart strong. High levels of insulin wreak havoc on the heart—a big concern for those with diabetes. "Elevated insulin triggers a bevy of heart disease risk factors," says Michael Zemel, PhD, chairman of the department of nutrition at the University of Tennessee in Knoxville. Dr. Zemel reviewed the connections between the glycemic index and heart disease for a scientific journal. He found that they include high blood pressure, increased fat storage, high triglycerides (a type of blood fat), and lower levels of HDL (the good cholesterol). Once again, low-GI foods appear to be the R_x. In the Nurses' Health Study, those women eating diets with the most carbohydrates from high-GI foods were nearly twice as likely to develop heart disease.

What Diabetes Experts Say

While organizations in other countries, such as the Canadian Diabetes Association, Australia's International Diabetes Institute, and the World Health Organization, all recommend including low-GI foods as part of managing diabetes, the glycemic index gets only a brief mention in the most recent practice guidelines from the American Diabetes Association (ADA).

"At this point, we don't recommend the glycemic index, because not enough is known. And there's no evidence that this method is better than the standard approach of counting carbohydrates," explains Marian Parrot, MD, vice president of clinical affairs for the ADA. Although Dr. Parrot agrees that the GI is "not harmful" and that "nothing is wrong with the science," her main objection is that it's too complicated—people just can't be expected to remember and deal with all those numbers. And in fact, a substantial group of health experts agree that although the glycemic index may prove useful someday, it is "not ready for prime time."

But in response, Dr. Rendell of Creighton Diabetes Center believes they are being overly cautious. "The authorities in the field are too

Surprisingly, sweet potatoes raise blood sugar much less than regular potatoes.

hung up on arithmetic," he says. "For instance, they bring up the fact that carrots have a high GI, so they're afraid people will stop eating carrots." But GI experts never advise avoiding high-GI foods that are low-calorie vegetables or fruits. "If high-GI foods such as carrots are also low in calories, you'd have to eat pounds of them to make much of an impact on blood sugar," says the University of Toronto's Dr. Wolever, coauthor of *The Glucose Revolution*.

He recommends targeting those high-GI foods that are also high in calories, such as baked goods, highly refined breakfast cereals, and potatoes. Start to replace them with lower-GI foods, such as trading in bagels for 100% stone-ground whole wheat bread, instant rice for barley, or cornflakes for All-Bran. "Switching to these low-GI starches," says Dr. Wolever, "can make a tremendous difference in your health."

For practical tips to start using the GI today, see "Six Secrets to Make the Glycemic Index Work for You" on p. 47.

CHAPTER 8

Easy Ways to Cook Healthier

Use these simple cooking tricks to make eating well easy—and delicious!

When you're used to eating certain foods and preparing them a certain way, making healthy changes can seem like a difficult task. But it really isn't! You don't have to completely change the types of food you eat and the way you cook to eat more healthfully. Simple adjustments such as substituting lower-fat versions of ingredients for higher-fat ones can make a big difference in how healthy you eat without sacrificing flavor.

Here's just one example: Use evaporated fat-free milk instead of heavy cream, and save more than 600 calories and nearly 90 g of fat per cup! Keep reading for a complete list of fat- and calorie-saving cooking swaps. These simple switches will make healthy eating easier than you ever thought it could be!

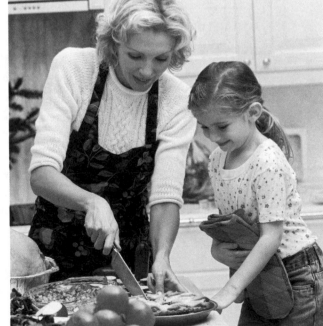

‖ Easy Fixes to Make Any Recipe Healthier

It's amazing how many calories and how much fat you can trim from recipes just by making small changes. Here are some ingredient substitutions to use in your favorite recipes.

Instead of	Use	Calories Saved	Fat Saved (g)
DAIRY PRODUCTS			
4 oz Cheddar cheese	4 oz reduced-fat Cheddar cheese (less than 5 g fat per oz)	171	25
	or 4 oz fat-free Cheddar cheese	293	38
4 oz feta cheese	2 oz feta cheese + 2 oz fat-free cottage cheese	115	12
4 oz chèvre (goat cheese)	2 oz chèvre + 2 oz fat-free ricotta cheese	160	16
8 oz cream cheese	8 oz light cream cheese	305	39
	or 8 oz fat-free cream cheese	588	79
	or 8 oz fat-free ricotta cheese	629	79
1 cup heavy cream	1 cup evaporated fat-free milk	621	87
1 cup sour cream	1 cup fat-free sour cream	347	48
	or 1 cup fat-free plain yogurt	366	48
	or 1 cup pureed fat-free cottage cheese + 1 tablespoon lemon juice	349	48
1 cup whole milk	1 cup fat-free milk	64	8
FATS AND OILS			
½ cup oil (for baking)	½ cup applesauce	911	109
	or ½ cup applesauce + ¼ cup buttermilk	912	108
	or ½ cup baby food prunes	799	109
½ cup oil (for marinades and salad dressings)	½ cup defatted chicken broth	945	109
	or ½ cup unsweetened pineapple juice	894	109
½ cup margarine or butter (for baking)	¼ cup reduced-calorie margarine (40% fat)	421	48
	or ½ cup applesauce	760	92
	or ¼ cup applesauce + ¼ cup buttermilk	761	91
	or ½ cup baby food prunes	681	92
½ cup margarine or butter (for icings)	½ cup marshmallow creme	392	92
2 tablespoons oil (for sautéing)	2 tablespoons defatted broth	236	27
	or 2 tablespoons unsweetened pineapple juice	223	27

Instead of	Use	Calories Saved	Fat Saved (g)
MEATS, POULTRY, FISH, AND EGGS			
1 lb ground beef (80% lean)	1 lb lean ground beef (95% lean)	350	27
	or 1 lb ground turkey breast	853	91
	or 1 lb ground turkey	268	32
	or 1 lb ground chicken	767	73
	or 1 lb ground chicken breast	811	89
	or 1 lb ground pork tenderloin	761	80
3 slices pork bacon (¾ oz total)	3 slices turkey bacon (¾ oz total)	42	5
3 oz roasted chicken thigh (with skin)	3 oz roasted chicken breast (without skin)	70	10
6½ oz canned oil-packed tuna	6½ oz canned water-packed tuna	124	14
1 whole egg	2 egg whites	41	5
MISCELLANEOUS			
1 cup chocolate	1 cup chocolate chips	215	15
	or ⅔ cup chocolate chips	286	20
	or ½ cup chocolate chips	430	30
1 oz unsweetened chocolate	3 tablespoons unsweetened cocoa powder	103	12
1 cup shredded coconut	½ cup shredded coconut	176	12
	or 1 teaspoon coconut flavoring	337	24
4 oz sliced olives	2 oz sliced olives	73	8
1 cup condensed canned cream soup	1 cup condensed canned 99% fat-free cream soup	112	13
1 cup sugar	¾ cup sugar	192	0
1 cup walnuts	½ cup walnuts	385	37

TAKE CONTROL: Grill and Bake

Automatically slim down your meals by using low-fat cooking methods such as grilling and baking instead of frying. Grilling intensifies flavors like no other cooking method can, because the high heat of the grill concentrates the food's tastes. And baking at high heat creates results similar to deep-frying, but without nearly as much fat. Try this with potatoes and breaded chicken, meats, and seafood.

CHAPTER 9

Eat Out without Guilt

Implement some smart strategies, and you can order up at almost any restaurant

Think eating out is a forbidden fantasy if you have diabetes? Well we have great news for you: Go ahead and book a table at your favorite Italian eatery. Grab lunch away from your desk—even at the drive-thru!

"People with diabetes can choose to eat healthfully and enjoy themselves in about 99% of all restaurants—but the operative word is *choose,*" says Hope S. Warshaw, RD, CDE, a

registered dietitian and certified diabetes educator based in Alexandria, VA, and author of *The Restaurant Companion: A Guide to Healthier Eating Out* (Surrey Books, 1995) and *Guide to Healthier Restaurant Eating* (American Diabetes Association, 1998). "Once you recognize the pitfalls of restaurant meals and learn a few simple strategies to manage them, you can do it."

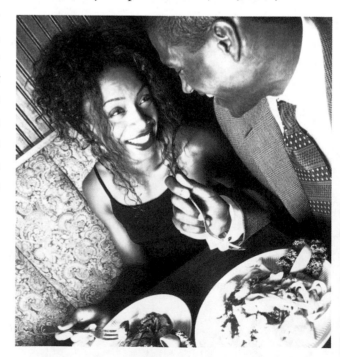

‖ Resist Temptation

The pitfalls are pretty obvious: Supersize portions with lots of hidden fat. The bottomless breadbasket and its tempting sidekick, the butter plate. The all-you-can-eat buffet. And your own habits and expectations. "If you eat out four times a week, but think of every meal as a special occasion, you're likely to give yourself license to not choose healthy meals and to overeat," Warshaw notes.

But with our plan, you can take control of what happens when someone else does the cooking. So you can eat out and enjoy great food, all the while knowing that you're still keeping your weight and blood sugar under control!

‖ Modify Your Mindset

Before you ever step foot into a restaurant, you have to make some changes to the way you think about eating out. Your first order of business is to begin thinking about limiting portions, avoiding excess fat, and ordering a meal that balances protein (usually meat or beans), carbohydrates (fruits, vegetables, dairy products, and grains), and fats. This will help most people with diabetes—and those at high risk for it—control blood sugar and avoid weight gain, or even lose unwanted pounds, says Terry Maratos-Flier, MD, associate professor of medicine at Harvard University Medical School and head of the obesity section at the Joslin Diabetes Center in Boston.

TAKE CONTROL: Call a Strategy Session

If you use insulin or another medication to help control blood sugar, discuss your dining out strategies with your dietitian so she can help you tailor your doses to specific foods and special situations, such as a delayed meal.

Here are three health goals that will help guide your menu choices.

Make weight loss your objective. If you need to, paring off pounds—even as few as 5 to 10—can have a positive impact on the quality of life of a person with diabetes. If you're having trouble imagining which foods will help you manage diabetes, just stick with lower-fat foods and smaller portion sizes, which can help you lose weight. Many restaurants even offer special selections or "light" entrées for people trying to slim down.

Find the right meal plan. Talk with your doctor and/or a dietitian who is a certified diabetes educator about a personalized plan to balance your intake of protein, carbohydrates, and fats to keep blood sugar as controlled as possible on a daily basis. (Ask about an exercise regimen too.) Some health insurance programs will even cover visits to a nutritionist.

"You might want to carry a card with your basic meal plan in your wallet to help guide you in making choices in a restaurant," advises Carolyn Leontos, RD, CDE, associate professor of nutrition at the University of Nevada in Reno and author of *What to Eat When You Get Diabetes*. "Or you can take some restaurant menus to your nutritionist so she can help you map out good meal choices."

Hire an official advisor: Give a dietitian the menus from your favorite eateries, and ask her what's okay to order.

Cutting Servings Down to Size

Looking to eat less? Here are three tricks for taming those gargantuan restaurant portions.

Order half "to go." "If you're the kind of person who will keep on eating if the food is left in front of you, ask the server to have the kitchen staff wrap half of your meal before it's served," suggests Amy Peterson Campbell, RD, CDE, of the Joslin Diabetes Center in Boston. Or, if you trust yourself, just ask the server to bring a take-out box with your order, and pack up half before you dig in. Built-in bonus: You've got lunch or dinner for tomorrow.

Share an entrée. "Here in Boston, there's a pasta chain where portions could easily feed three for dinner," Campbell notes. "One of the best strategies there, and elsewhere, is to share a meal with someone else, and order a salad or a plain vegetable side dish to round out the meal." In a steak house, you might order a steak, salad, and baked potato, while your dinner companion orders just the salad and baked potato and shares your steak. At an Italian restaurant, mix and match a pasta meal with a chicken-and-vegetable dish.

Try the "small plates" approach. Instead of a big entrée, order an appetizer plus soup and/or some vegetable-based side dishes. "When ordering, think in terms of what you can realistically eat," suggests Hope S. Warshaw, RD, CDE, a registered dietitian based in Alexandria, VA. "It may seem like a small thing, but try it—you'll probably be satisfied."

Choose a "safe" meal. "When you're eating just to fuel up, deciding on a balanced, predetermined meal before you even enter a restaurant can take the worry out of eating out," says Amy Peterson Campbell, RD, CDE, a registered dietitian with the Joslin Diabetes Center in Boston and author of *16 Myths of a Diabetic Diet.* Ask your nutritionist or physician for help in choosing an entrée, side dishes, and drink that work for you. "A businesswoman with diabetes told me she was on the road all day and had to eat lunch out. Rather than try to figure out what she could eat from a new restaurant menu every day, she settled on a basic meal that isn't too high in calories or fat: broiled fish, a baked potato, and salad with dressing on the side," says Campbell. "She can order it anywhere."

Strategize Before You're Seated

Maximize the pleasure of the restaurant experience, minimize temptation, and ensure that you'll get the meal you want—by strategizing before you even make a reservation. Here's how.

Adjust the frequency. "Having one or two higher-fat, higher-calorie meals a week, such as a restaurant meal, isn't usually a problem for most people with diabetes," says Campbell. "If you tend to eat out more than that, you may want to cut back so that you can enjoy one or two restaurant meals a week without putting on pounds or throwing your blood sugar off."

Ask for stats. Many fast-food outlets and restaurant chains make nutritional information about menu items available—at the restaurant, on the Internet, or by mail. Just ask. "The more you know, the healthier your choices can be," Warshaw notes. If you can't find anything suitable at one place, try another.

Know thyself. The best single strategy? "People need to identify their own issues and problems while eating out, then find solutions," Warshaw says. "This is true whether you have diabetes or not. If a breadbasket on the table is a problem, see what works for you: Getting it off the table? Taking one piece and setting the rest out of arm's reach? You'll have to see."

Here's more advice: "By the same token, if you like Chinese or Thai food and feel tempted by all those high-fat appetizers that your friends are having, try ordering a healthier broth-based soup so you won't be the only one without an appetizer,"

says Warshaw. "And if you can't resist finishing that big bowl of pasta at the local Italian spot, consider ordering something entirely different instead, and just completely remove the temptation. Or see if you can get the pasta in an appetizer size."

Use your imagination. Before you arrive at the restaurant, help yourself avoid temptation and sidestep the danger of feeling deprived by visualizing yourself enjoying a healthy meal, talking with your companions, and feeling full and satisfied. Even if you're just zipping in and out of the drive-thru, imagine the hamburger, salad, and diet drink you'll enjoy—so you're ready to say "no thanks" to the fries and shake when placing your order. "A plain hamburger has about 350 calories, which is fine," says Dr. Maratos-Flier. "But add regular fries, and you'll consume an additional 600 calories."

Forbidden Foods You Can Order

Chocolate cake? A glass of chardonnay? Ice cream? A beer? Strawberry shortcake? Scotch and soda?

Once considered off-limits for people with diabetes, desserts and alcoholic beverages are now viewed by experts as occasional treats that can be worked into many meal plans, says nutritionist Amy Peterson Campbell, RD, CDE, of the Joslin Diabetes Center in Boston. "It's an enduring myth that you can't have a drink or a sweet ending to a meal," she says. "What people need to do is find out how these foods affect their blood sugar levels, and then plan accordingly. Some people may still find that they're too disruptive." But you may be among the many who *can* work in a little treat now and then. Here's what you need to know.

Sweets: Plan ahead, and forego having both a carbohydrate and a fat serving at the same meal to leave room for dessert, advises Campbell. "Then consider splitting with someone else. Many desserts are quite large these days." Later, use your blood sugar monitor to see how your body reacts, and adjust your eating accordingly next time you dine.

Alcohol: "One or two drinks is usually fine for most people with diabetes," Campbell says. "Choosing wine, light beer, or a hard liquor such as scotch or gin is better than a sugary mixed drink such as a margarita or a piña colada." If you control diabetes with medication, talk with your doctor first; alcohol can lower blood sugar.

Stay Strong All Meal Long

Okay, your pager went off. The hostess led you to your table. You have the menu in hand. You're salivating. What you do next is going to determine the state of your blood sugar, your body weight, and, to some degree, your future health. Here's how to stick to your guns and still enjoy your meal.

Divide and conquer huge portions. Supersize lunches. "Biggie" boxes of fries. Huge heaps of pasta. Bucket-size cups, brimming with sugary soft drinks. "Oversize portions are one of the big reasons more and more Americans are overweight—and increasingly at risk for diabetes," Dr. Maratos-Flier says. "I'd say serving size is the number one thing to deal with when eating out. Too many bites equals too many calories." (See "Cutting Servings Down to Size" on p. 58 for ideas on how to keep giant meals from getting the best of you.)

Uncover hidden fat. Creamy and flavorful, moist and satisfying—and loaded with calories— fat is everywhere on restaurant menus. "Luckily, you can order flavorful, lower-fat versions of many entrées and even appetizers by asking a few questions and making simple requests," Leontos notes. For starters, suggests Warshaw, be alert for high-fat ingredients, including butter, oil, cream, and sour

(See "Cutting Servings Down to Size" on p. 58)

> **TAKE CONTROL: Open Your Mouth**
>
> Need low-fat salad dressing? Want to know how large that entrée really is? Wonder how much fat is in the chef's special sauce? Just ask. Celebrities special-order all the time, so why shouldn't you?

cream; high-fat foods, such as cheese, avocado, and sausage; and high-fat cooking techniques, such as frying, sautéing, and broiling with butter.

Request simple switches. It's often easy to bring down a meal's calorie count by making a few substitutions. If you can, request high-fat sauces on the side, skip the cheese on made-to-order items (such as sandwiches and some Mexican dishes), and ask to have fish and poultry broiled with either no fat or minimal amounts, says Leontos. And choose reduced-calorie or reduced-fat dressings and mustard for salads and sandwiches. "If you feel comfortable, tell your server that you have diabetes and need to watch what you eat," she suggests. If you don't want to share that info, just say you're trying to eat a healthy meal. She may be able to suggest healthier options that you hadn't even considered.

Focus on "good fats." People with diabetes are at higher risk for heart disease, so controlling cholesterol is important. Focus on eating less saturated fats (found in meats, cheese, whole milk, and full-fat yogurt and sour cream) and less

Try, try again: Do whatever it takes to identify your weaknesses, then work around them. If a breadbasket on the table is a problem, try sending it back. Or take one piece, and set the rest out of reach.

trans fats (found in fried and processed foods). Choosing olive or canola oil (with monounsaturated fats that help preserve levels of good HDL cholesterol) is a healthier strategy, Leontos notes.

Make Sure Your Plan's Working

The last step in dining out with diabetes is paying attention to the effects on your blood sugar and your weight. Here's one of the best ways to do just that.

Check yourself. When you dine out, keep notes about what you eat, and take notice of how it affects your blood sugar levels when you check later. This type of regular monitoring will help you see how different foods and cuisines affect your blood sugar so you can make better choices in the future, Leontos says. It will help you see if your efforts are working, or whether you need to adjust your meal plan, lose more weight, or consider medication, says Dr. Maratos-Flier. Monitor your levels as prescribed by your doctor—up to four times a day if you have diabetes, two or three times a week if you're insulin-resistant.

CHAPTER 10

Eat Your Way to a Healthier Weight

Losing just a few pounds will put you in charge of your diabetes!

Here's some news that should motivate you to take off a few pounds: Losing as little as 10 lb can not only make you look better and boost your energy, but it can also help improve your insulin function and lower your blood sugar levels. And that puts you in better control of your diabetes. If you've got early diabetes, or impaired glucose tolerance, a loss of 5% of your body weight (that's just 8 lb if you weigh 160, for example) can lower your risk of getting full-blown diabetes by a whopping 80 to 100%!

Now that you know how little you have to lose to reap big advantages over diabetes, here are some strategies you can combine with your healthy eating and exercise plans that will ensure weight loss success.

Eating Strategies That Work

Food grouping programs such as the Diabetes Food Exchange System will definitely help you eat a more balanced diet and keep portions under control, both of which are key to weight loss (and good diabetes management). But there are some other easy guidelines that may help you if you're trying to take off pounds. We uncovered these other key principles to eating smart for weight loss from people who have lost weight—and kept it off. Here's what really works.

Always eat when you're hungry. The people in the National Weight Control Registry eat an average of five meals a day. The fact is, most

Three Easy Weight Loss Goals

Start off your weight loss plan by aiming for the three small diet goals below. You can achieve each goal with one little switch, as our examples show. Then watch your weight loss success grow from there!

1. Lose 8 lb.
To drop 8 lb in 1 year, do one of these:
➤ Have flavored seltzer instead of a 12-oz can of Coke or Pepsi—four times a week (about 150 fewer calories a day).
➤ Have a 1-oz bag of pretzels instead of a doughnut for coffee break—5 days a week (about 120 fewer calories a day).
➤ Have a Nutri-Grain Strawberries & Creme Twist instead of a Frosted Strawberry Pop-Tart for breakfast—every day (about 75 fewer calories a day).

2. Eat less fat.
To cut total daily fat intake by 22 g and saturated fat by 6 g (one-half of the maximum fat for women, one-third for men), do one of these:
➤ Have a turkey sandwich with two tomato slices instead of two Cheddar cheese slices.
➤ Have 1 cup tapioca pudding instead of 1 cup Häagen-Dazs ice cream.
➤ Have a Subway 6" Roast Beef Sub instead of a McDonald's Quarter Pounder with Cheese.

3. Get more fiber.
Fiber helps to block the fat your body absorbs. To add 6 to 8 g fiber— one-quarter of the fiber you need in a day—do one of these:
➤ Have 1 cup Raisin Bran cereal (8 g) instead of 1 cup Cocoa Puffs (0 g).
➤ Have ½ cup baked beans (7 g) instead of ½ cup pasta salad (1 g).
➤ Have 1 large apple (7 g) instead of a fruit roll-up (0 g).
➤ Have 1 cup lentil soup (7 g) instead of 1 cup chicken with rice soup (1 g).

folks need to eat every 2 to 4 hours. Otherwise, we override our built-in mechanism that tells us when we're hungry and when we've had enough. We're starved, so then we overeat. Learn to recognize your hunger cues— grumbly tummy, energy crash, irritability—and eat in response to them.

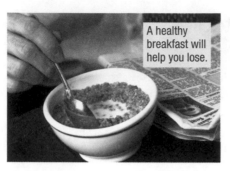

A healthy breakfast will help you lose.

Naturally slim people eat only when they're truly hungry, according to Vicki Hansen, MSW, coauthor of *The Seven Secrets of Slim People*. These lucky folks eat differently than the rest of us. All of us were born with this ability. But we let appetite, cravings, and years of conditioning to clean our plates short-circuit our hunger mechanism. The fact is, denying hunger and skipping meals always backfire.

Stop when you're full. Your body tells you when it has had enough to eat. But the signs are subtle. You may need to relearn how to recognize these signals. One way is to eat slowly. It takes your body about 20 minutes to feel the food you eat. If you eat too quickly, you'll eat right past the point of being satisfied, and you'll eat too much. Another trick is to wear clothing with zippered waistbands instead of the elastic kind. Elasticized skirts and slacks are very forgiving, but something snug around your waist will signal you to stop eating as it tightens up.

Eat a good breakfast. Breakfast helps you avoid overeating later in the day. Go for foods that have some protein and a little fat in addition to carbohydrates and sugar. They will give you the energy you need to make it through the morning. Good choices are whole grain cereal with 1% milk, eggs and toast, or a fruity breakfast smoothie. Beware of sugary breakfast foods such as kids' cereals and Danish. While initially satisfying, these are out of your system in about 30 minutes, leaving you hungry for more.

Count calories, not just fat. Sure, fat has more calories than protein or carbohydrate foods (9 calories per gram versus 4 for protein and carbohydrate foods). But that doesn't mean that eating only low-fat foods will help you lose weight. Research done at the University of Vermont in Burlington showed that there's more to weight loss than counting fat grams. One group of dieters was asked to restrict their fat to 22 to 26 g per day but not to count calories. Another group was asked to count calories but not fat. After 6 months, the calorie counters lost more than twice as much weight as those who restricted fat. Why? One reason is the incredible number of low-fat products on the market that are not low in calories. By only counting fat grams, you could be taking in more calories than you need.

Fill up on fiber. Combined with a good supply of water, fiber-rich foods are a dieter's

---

TAKE CONTROL: Combine Diet with a Little Exercise

The easiest way to lose weight is to combine a healthy diet with some exercise. If you want to lose a pound a week (a healthy weight loss rate), create a 500-calorie deficit each day. For instance, exercise off 300 calories (that's a 3- to 4-mile walk or an exercise class), and cut back on what you eat by 200 calories.

Find Your Target Weight Range

Use this chart to help determine your weight goals. Remember that these numbers represent a range that is appropriate for men and women. They are not absolutes, so use them only as a guide. Find your height in the left column, and move across the chart to find your weight range in pounds. If you have a small frame, you should be at the lower end of the range. If you've got a larger frame, the upper end is acceptable.

Height	Male	Female
4'8"	74–90	72–88
4'9"	79–97	77–94
4'10"	85–103	81–99
4'11"	90–110	86–105
5'	95–117	90–110
5'1"	101–123	95–116
5'2"	106–130	99–121
5'3"	112–136	104–127
5'4"	117–143	108–132
5'5"	122–150	113–138
5'6"	128–156	117–143
5'7"	133–163	122–149
5'8"	139–169	126–154
5'9"	144–176	131–160
5'10"	149–183	135–165
5'11"	155–189	140–171
6'	160–196	144–176
6'1"	166–202	149–182
6'2"	171–209	153–187
6'3"	176–216	158–193
6'4"	182–222	162–198
6'5"	187–229	167–204
6'6"	193–235	171–209

dream. They're filling and come packaged with lots of vitamins, minerals, and other helpful plant nutrients. What are the best sources of fiber? Whole grains such as cereals, whole wheat bread, and brown rice; watery vegetables such as salad greens, tomatoes, zucchini, green beans, and broccoli; and fruits such as apples and oranges.

Look at portion sizes. We're used to seeing our plates full. But if you're eating from a huge dinner plate, it's probably too much food. Portion sizes are especially important for controlling blood sugar. In addition to following the serving guidelines on p. 32, try using smaller plates. Keep in mind that a cup is about the size of your fist, and a portion of meat or fish is about the size of a deck of cards. If you're going out for fast food, choose a kids' meal in place of the "Super Combo." You'll save an average of about 438 calories per meal at most restaurants. Having a salad? Eat as much as you want—but be sparing with what goes on top.

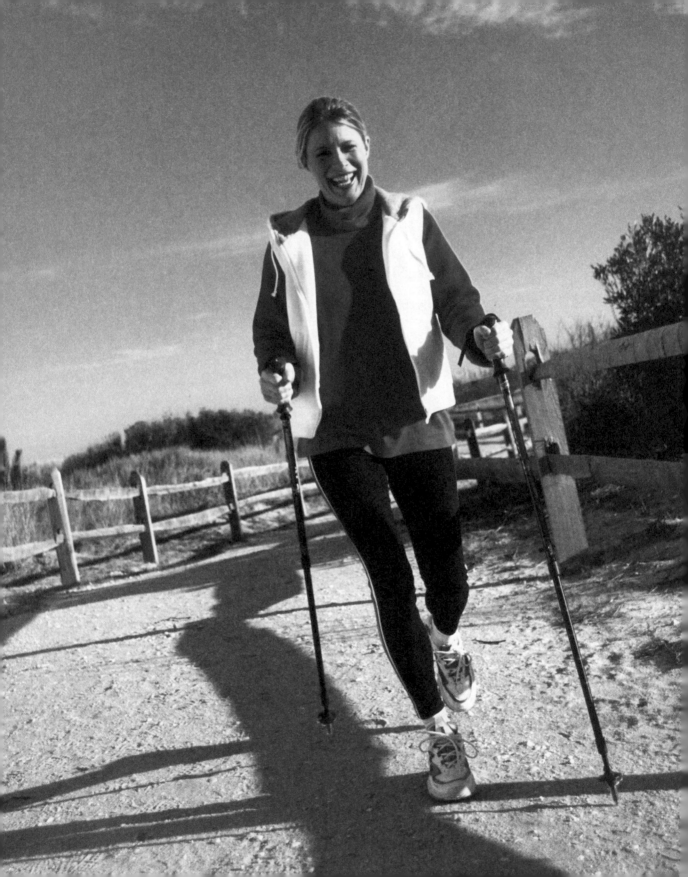

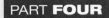

PART FOUR

Exercise Prescriptions for Diabetes

Get moving—even just a little bit—and watch your blood sugar improve

CHAPTER 11

7 Steps to a Safe Workout

Make sure you have a problem-free workout with these simple tips

Exercise should be a regular prescription if you have diabetes. Why? It keeps your weight under control, which is especially important with this disease. It helps to control blood sugar, which reduces the risk of diabetes-related complications, such as nerve and eye damage, and protects against heart disease, which diabetes sufferers are at increased risk of developing. Exercise also improves heart function and bloodflow, which can help reduce the risk of circulatory problems.

While you need to make exercise a regular part of your routine if you have diabetes, you also have to take a few extra steps to ensure a safe and rewarding workout. For instance, you need to pay special attention to your feet and watch for signs of high blood sugar. Here are all the details you need to know.

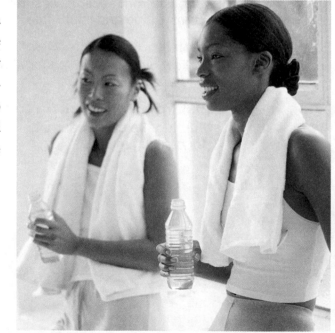

‖ How to Play It Safe

1. Check your blood sugar first. Under 100 mg/dl? Eat a carbohydrate snack (such as a banana or whole wheat bagel) before working out. Between 250 and 300 mg/dl? Test for ketones, by-products created when the body breaks down fat because it doesn't have enough insulin. If the results are positive, don't exercise. Higher than 300 mg/dl? Don't exercise.

2. Inject insulin into your abdomen, instead of your arm or thigh, to prevent absorption difficulties.

3. Look out for insulin reaction warning signs. If you feel faint, dizzy, or confused, stop immediately and have some OJ, nondiet soda, or glucose tablets. An insulin reaction can occur during your workout or at any time in the 12 hours that follow it.

4. Drink plenty of water. Dehydration can raise blood sugar. Take in fluids before, during, and after you exercise.

5. Identify yourself. A diabetes identification bracelet or shoe tag should be clearly visible, especially if you're exercising alone.

6. Protect your eyes. If you have retinopathy, avoid exercises that significantly raise heart rate and blood pressure (such as heavy lifting and jogging) or that put you in an upside-down position (such as some yoga moves).

7. Do a postworkout foot check. Impaired sensation in your feet may prevent you

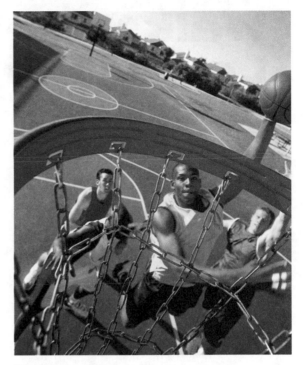

Exercise helps control blood sugar, sheds pounds, and protects against heart disease.

from feeling an injury. Left untreated, it could cause more serious problems. If you have peripheral neuropathy, avoid exercises that are hard on your feet, such as running and tennis.

TAKE CONTROL: Tell Your Teammates

If you're working out with others, tell them about your condition and how they can help you if a problem arises. If you work out alone, let someone know what you'll be doing, where you'll be, and when you'll be done. (This is good advice for nondiabetics too!)

CHAPTER 12

Walk Your Way to Lower Blood Sugar

Why walking is the ultimate workout for people with diabetes—plus a complete plan to get started

If you're looking for a type of exercise that will give you all the diabetes-controlling benefits and is also convenient and easy to do, walking is the perfect choice. There's no equipment required (except a good pair of walking shoes), you can do it indoors or outside, and you can alter the pace to fit what's most comfortable for you.

Haven't exercised in awhile? That's not a problem, because we've included a 4-week beginner's walking plan on p. 72. This regimen will ease you into a walking routine and get you up to speed before you know it. Whether you choose to follow this plan or create your own workout schedule, you'll feel great knowing all the good those walks are doing for your body!

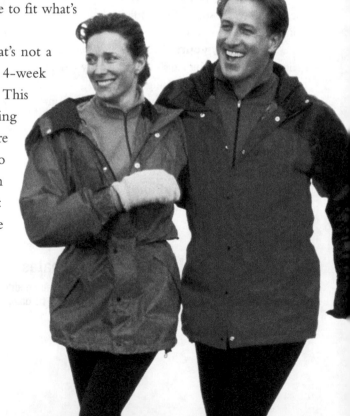

The Benefits of Walking

The combination of a healthy diet and regular physical activity such as walking can help you slim down—an important benefit, because overweight is a major risk factor for diabetes.

But exercise fights diabetes in ways other than weight loss. Studies are just starting to show the preventive power of fitness. The famed Nurses' Health Study, for example, found that women who worked up a sweat more than once a week reduced their risk of developing diabetes by 30%. And Chinese researchers determined that people with high blood sugar who engaged in moderate exercise (and made other lifestyle changes) were 40% less likely to develop full-blown diabetes. "It wasn't really vigorous exercise either," notes Richard Eastman, MD, former director of the diabetes division of the National Institute of Diabetes and Digestive and Kidney Diseases in Bethesda, MD.

How Walking Helps

Why does walking have such protective effects? Besides helping you get rid of extra pounds, it actually increases the number of insulin receptors on your cells. Insulin helps blood sugar move into cells, where it needs to go. Otherwise, it just sloshes around in your bloodstream, gumming up the blood vessel walls. If you've already been diagnosed with diabetes, regular walking can help control the progression of the disease. People who take insulin may be able to reduce the amount of medication they need, because physical activity enables their body to use insulin more efficiently.

"Walking Got Me off Medication"

Two years ago, George Coman, 56, thought he was dying when he stumbled into the Joslin Diabetes Center in Boston. His blood sugar levels were eight times the norm, and he was diagnosed with diabetes. On his doctor's advice, George started walking 2½ miles 6 days a week. Then he increased to walking/running 3½ miles and began lifting weights. In 1 year, he lost 40 lb, dropped his glucose levels, and no longer needed any medications.

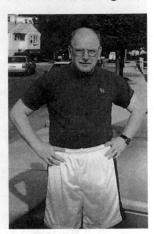

As a bonus, regular walking can help keep your brain sharp. Scientists have observed that older people with diabetes sometimes have problems thinking clearly. In one study, physical activity appeared to stimulate just the type of brain activity that had become impaired. Exactly what it is about physical activity that revs up the brain hasn't been determined. But some experts theorize that exercise-related brain activity could be part of the reason why some folks say they are able to solve sticky problems while they're ticking off minutes and miles on their treadmill.

For all of these reasons, walking may be one of the best diabetes therapies around.

The Beginner's Walking Plan

This program is designed to ease you into a regular walking routine. By starting out slowly, you'll enjoy it more, build your confidence, and reduce your risk of injury. After about 2 weeks, your walks will feel easier, because your heart will be fitter and your legs will be stronger. By week 4, you'll be up to 30 minutes 5 days a week—well within the amount of walking recommended to help control blood sugar.

	Duration	Frequency	Intensity	Speed
Week 1	10 min	3 days	moderate*	whatever is comfortable
Week 2	15 min	4 days	moderate*	as if you're in a hurry; after walking for 10 minutes, you should have covered more distance than you did last week
Week 3	20 min	5 days	moderate*	as if you're in a hurry
Week 4	30 min	5 days	moderate*	as if you're in a hurry

*enough to get your heart pumping, but not enough to leave you out of breath

Make Walks Work for You

Before you begin a walking program, check with your doctor, especially if you already have diabetes. He can tell you whether you need to take any special precautions when you work out.

According to Gerald Bernstein, MD, former president of the American Diabetes Association, you must exercise for at least 30 minutes three times a week to enhance your body's use of insulin. If your goal is to lose weight, however, you would do well to walk five to seven times each week. Of course, you'll want to work up to that level slowly, especially if you have been sedentary. (See "The Beginner's Walking Plan" above.) If you skip a day, don't try to make up for

it by walking twice as fast or twice as far during your next workout. Vigorous exercise can actually cause blood sugar to rise, especially in people who have insulin deficiency.

If you have diabetes, the timing of your walks can help regulate your blood sugar levels. People with type 2 diabetes may benefit from exercising before meals, which helps control appetite and promote weight loss. And for those with type 1, it's best not to exercise on an empty stomach. These folks should plan to walk about an hour or so after a meal, when blood sugar levels are at their highest.

There are times when exercise can send blood sugar plummeting.

This reaction is most common among people who use insulin. Ask your doctor how much exercise you can tolerate before you need to replenish your store of carbohydrates. And carry a healthy snack—such as a piece of fresh fruit, dried fruit, or some peanuts or trail mix—with you for just this purpose.

‖ Warm Up First

It's critically important to warm up and cool down during every workout. Start by strolling for 3 to 5 minutes, then stretch key walking muscles: your calves, quadriceps (the muscles on the front of your thighs), and hamstrings (the muscles on the back of your thighs).

It's also good to stretch the sides of your

You must exercise for at least 30 minutes three times a week to enhance your body's use of insulin.

torso, shoulders, and arms. (Just be sure to stretch both sides evenly.) Hold each stretch for 20 to 30 seconds during your warm-up. At the end of your walk, cool down by walking slowly for 5 minutes, then repeat the stretches, this time holding each stretch a little longer (about 45 to 60 seconds).

Follow these smart stretching tips:

• Stretch to the point that you feel tension—not pain—then hold the stretch there.

Put Your Feet to the Test

People with diabetes need to be extravigilant about foot care. A common side effect of the disease is a loss of sensation (called diabetic neuropathy) that can allow minor injuries to turn into major problems. "If you can't feel a blister, you may not treat it properly," explains Linda Haas, RN, CDE (certified diabetes educator), president of health care and education at the American Diabetes Association. "The wound can become infected, which may lead to ulcerations and even amputation."

Determine your risk. There's a home test kit that can help you find out if your feet are at risk for injury. Offered free of charge by the Lower Extremity Amputation Prevention (LEAP) program, the kit contains a reusable monofilament (something like a fishing line) that you press against your foot. If you can't feel the monofilament, you may be losing sensation, and you should see your doctor. In one study, the monofilament test was accurate 87% of the time.

How to order. To get your kit from the Bureau of Primary Health Care, write to Free Filament, LEAP Program, P.O. Box 2910, Merrifield, VA 22116. Or call toll-free (888) ASK-HRSA (275-4772), or go online at http://bphc.hrsa.gov/leap.

In addition to using the monofilament test, you should continue to visually inspect your feet for blisters on a daily basis and especially after walking.

• Hold a stretch gently and smoothly. Don't bounce.

• Stretch both sides of your body evenly.

Take Care of Your Feet

If you've been diagnosed with diabetes, your doctor has likely told you the importance of taking care of your feet. Not only is it important, it's imperative. Any small blister or callus can turn into a dangerous situation. Unfortunately, people with diabetes often have difficulty feeling problems with their feet, because of nerve damage associated with the condition. To complicate matters, they're also more prone to infection. Even the slightest irritation left undetected and untreated can lead to major complications.

So if you're launching a walking program, do what you can to keep your feet healthy.

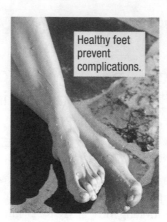

Healthy feet prevent complications.

Above all else, that means investing in comfortable socks and great-fitting walking shoes. Keep them free of rough spots and foreign particles to prevent irritation and injury. (For several good makes of shoes to choose from, see chapter 13: "The Best Shoes for Walking Workouts.")

Inspect your feet on a daily basis, and apply baby powder to keep them dry and to discourage the formation of blisters. If you notice any irritation or injury, consult a physician or podiatrist immediately—within 24 hours. (See "Put Your Feet to the Test" on p. 73 for more information about checking your feet.)

If there's any good to be found in diabetes, it's that the condition can motivate you to lead a healthy lifestyle that includes walking regularly. And that means not only better health and greater longevity but also increased enjoyment of life.

CHAPTER 13

The Best Shoes for Walking Workouts

Choose from seven styles that will keep your feet comfortable and injury-free

People with diabetes need to take special care of their feet, which means wearing shoes that don't rub and cause irritation such as ulcers. To avoid discomfort and continue walking your way to better blood sugar, you should have a shoe specific to the type of walking you'll be doing. Hitting some light trails? Try a trail walker. Plan to walk around your neighborhood? Choose a casual walking shoe.

"Sport-specific" shoes, whether for casual, serious, or trail walking, provide just the right construction to keep your feet stable, help them through the heel-to-toe motion of walking, support your weight properly, and ease the impact of walking mile after mile. In this chapter we review seven great styles to consider. Turn the page to find the perfect walking shoe for you!

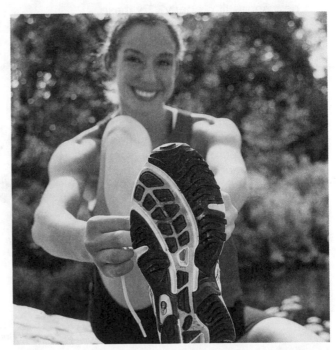

‖ For Fitness Walks

If you want to rack up serious walking mileage, here are four of our favorites. You can get these (or any style in this chapter) from The Walker's Warehouse at toll-free (888) 972-9255 or www.walkerswarehouse.com.

New Balance shoes come in many sizes and widths and can accommodate hard-to-fit feet. The **655** is geared to the fast-paced walker; it's very light, supportive, and flexible. It's got plenty of toe wiggle room and stabilizes your feet as you

New Balance 655.

Get the Perfect Fit

Looking for some tips to make sure your new shoes fit properly? Try these.

Make a template. Before you buy a new pair of shoes, trace your feet on a piece of paper, and cut out the shape—that's your template. If the template is wider than the sole of the shoe you're trying, look for a different size or brand for a better fit.

Wear your socks. When you try on shoes, be sure to wear the socks you'll wear on your fitness walks. These socks tend to take up more space and could force you into a different size.

Wait until day's end. To get your walking shoes to fit properly, wait till the end of the day to try them on, when your feet are their largest.

walk. It also provides ample cushioning and shock absorption. Mesh in the upper helps keep your feet cool while you're turning on the steam. It offers good traction for both indoor and outdoor walking. Price: $65. The 655 is widely available at retailers. To locate a dealer, go to www.newbalance.com.

Ryka's high-performance walking shoe, the **Doyenne,** offers special features that ensure motion stability. Designed for fast walkers, the Doyenne provides extra cushioning for the heel, so if you've ever had any twinges of heel pain, you might want to give this shoe a try. (Hint: Stretching your calf muscles also helps prevent certain kinds of heel pain.) The Doyenne has a synthetic upper with lots of mesh for breathability and a sporty look. It's very light and offers great flexibility. This shoe tends to run small, so try one size larger than is normal for you. Price: $70. To locate a dealer near you, visit www.ryka.com or call toll-free (888) 834-RYKA (7952).

Ryka Doyenne.

The **Saucony Grid Motion** is also a great shoe for serious walkers. Often recommended for people who overpronate—their heels tend to roll inward—this shoe supports your arches, holds your feet steady, and offers lots of great cushioning. The beveled heel and forefoot grooves help you move through the heel-to-

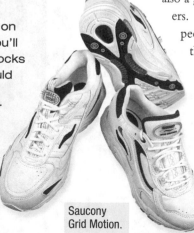

Saucony Grid Motion.

toe walking motion comfortably. Price: $70. For dealers, call (800) 365-7282, or go to www.saucony.com.

Avia 362.

The **Avia 362** is a good all-around walking shoe for both beginners and established walkers. This shoe offers lots of stability but doesn't feel quite as lightweight or flexible as the New Balance, Ryka, or Saucony styles listed above. The Avia 362 will help keep you from over-pronating, and it feels comfortable even if you have low arches. It features leather uppers and extra heel cushioning too. Since this shoe tends to run small, you might want to try a half-size larger than usual. Price: $55. To find a dealer, go to www.avia.com or call toll-free (888) 855-2842.

For Trail Walks

If you prefer wooded trails to tracks, city streets, or suburban neighborhoods, then you probably don't want a spanking-white walking shoe. What you do need is a little more traction and protec-

Timberland Spruce Pass.

tion, yet not quite a hiking boot. Our favorite "light trail" shoe is the **Timberland Spruce Pass,** a great off-road walking shoe for women.

This shoe is so light you'll barely notice you have it on, except for the great traction and motion control it gives you. Unlike some trail shoes, this one has plenty of flexibility, and the special foam liner keeps your feet nice and cool (and offers you a little extra protection from sticks and stones). Bonus: The color won't show the dirt! Price: $85. To locate a dealer near you, call (800) 445-5545, or visit www.timberland.com.

For Casual Walks

Want a slip-on shoe that's as comfy and supportive as a full-fledged walking shoe but doesn't look like one? Try the **Merrell Jungle Moc.** This shoe, made for both men and women, glides on like a bedroom slipper and feels just as luxurious. But what's surprising about the Jungle Moc is its stability. What's more, this shoe features an inner stretch band (called a gusset) that hugs your foot. The Jungle Moc also offers three other wonderful features: good traction, a footbed that matches the contours of your feet, and great cushioning. You can wear these funky-looking shoes while walking on level trails, shopping at the mall, or working on casual Fridays. It comes in several colors. Price: $65

Merrell Jungle Moc.

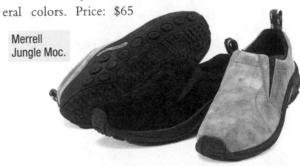

Control the Motion!

Besides comfort, if there's one feature that characterizes all of the shoes we've mentioned here, it's motion control. Proper motion control means that when you walk, your feet and ankles remain stable, moving from side to side very little. The more stability in your feet and ankles, the more efficiently you'll walk, and the less strain your ankles will suffer. Good stability also prevents overpronation and supination, which happen when your feet lean too far either inward or outward, respectively.

(men's and women's). For a dealer near you, call toll-free (888) 637-7001, or surf to www.merrellboot.com.

Wolky Hand.

‖ For the Office

If you like to walk during your lunch break but find most comfort shoes too casual for work, and most dress-up shoes too tight for comfort, check out the **Wolky** collection. Hailing from the Netherlands, Wolky shoes look like clogs, with the kind of roomy toe box that makes your piggies squeal for joy. Their anatomically shaped cork footbeds are light and shock absorbing, and they take on the shape of your feet as you wear them. The rocker bottom makes striding effortless, and handy Velcro closures make fitting them a breeze.

Wolky's styles are supercomfortable for work, as well as stable enough to take a casual walk break during the day without changing shoes. They're youthful and stylish but high enough off the ground to keep your trousers from dragging as you walk. One great choice is the **Hand,** a Mary Jane–style shoe in ultrasoft leather with a Velcro strap. Price: $110 to $130. To locate a dealer near you, call (800) WOLKY31 (965-5931), or visit their Web site at www.wolky.com.

CHAPTER 14

Flatten Your Belly to Beat Diabetes

Follow our 2-week plan for a trimmer middle and a healthier you

A flat belly does a lot more than make you look great in a bathing suit or jeans—it can actually save your life! Scientific research continues to show that a trim middle can protect you against several life-threatening diseases, including diabetes.

Unlike the fat on your thighs (which doesn't pose much of a health risk), the size of your belly is directly related to your risk of disease. In fact, women with the highest waist circumferences—36 inches or larger—were five times more likely to develop diabetes compared with those whose waistlines were about 26 inches, according to one study. But don't worry—our 2-week plan will help you rein in that belly bulge and take control of your diabetes in no time!

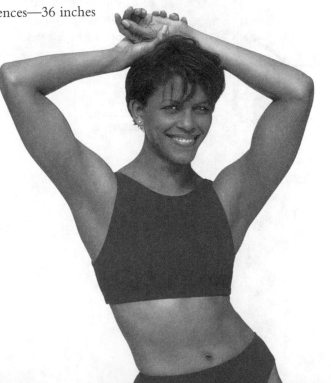

Why You Need a Smaller Waistline

Other studies show that a waistline of 32 inches (37 inches for men) or more may put you at greater risk for health problems. This is because fat inside the abdomen is more likely to release fatty acids into the liver than fat elsewhere on the body, says Henry S. Kahn, MD, associate professor of family and preventive medicine at Emory University School of Medicine in Atlanta. The result can be excessive amounts of insulin and cholesterol in the bloodstream.

In addition, abdominal fat appears to be related to insulin resistance, says Dr. Kahn. (That means your cells don't respond to insulin as they should. As a result, your blood sugar levels remain unusually high.) It's likely that over time, this resistance causes your body to stop producing insulin, resulting in diabetes.

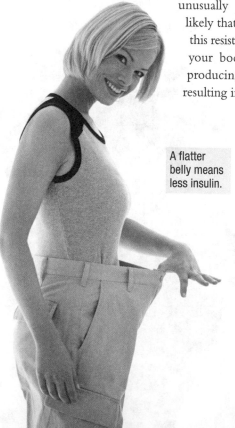

A flatter belly means less insulin.

TAKE CONTROL: Get Some Sleep
One of the best ways to fight stress—which may increase your belt size—is a good night's sleep. For better sleep, exercise daily, but avoid vigorous activity for at least 2 hours before bedtime.

But you don't have to let that happen. Our plan, backed by scientific research involving more than 100,000 people, will help you fight belly fat so that you can look fantastic, live longer, and control your diabetes. Get started today, and see results in 2 weeks!

Nine Steps to a Flatter Belly

We scoured the latest scientific research and talked to leading experts to find out the best ways to get your tummy in line. Here are nine that will take inches from your waistline—and help you prevent or take charge of diabetes.

1. Go (nearly) meatless. The best way to predict whether or not you'll need larger pants is to look at your plate. "Women who ate the most meat [more than seven servings a week] were 1½ times more likely to expand their waistlines than were women who ate two or less servings," says Dr. Kahn, referring to a 10-year study of nearly 80,000 people.

This doesn't mean that you have to give up meat: It's about moderation. "Few people in our study were vegetarians," Dr. Kahn says. "They just ate like they were." Limit yourself to one serving of meat every 2 or 3 days, and make up the difference with fruits and veggies—at least five a day, but aim for nine. "They act as protection from gaining weight," he says.

Size Up Your Belly

"You can get just as much information about your health risks from your abdominal circumference as you can from more complicated measurements, such as a calculated waist-to-hip ratio," says Robert J. Kuczmarski, DrPH, an epidemiologist at the National Center for Health Statistics in Hyattsville, MD. But your abdominal circumference isn't the same as your waist size. Here's how to get an accurate measurement.

1. First, use your thumb to feel for the point on your side (think of a line running from your armpit) where the top of your hipbone gives way to soft tissue. "For most people, this point is even with the belly button, but using the hipbone is more reliable," says Dr. Kuczmarski, who developed the standard.

2. Place your tape measure just above that bone, and loop it around your belly, being careful to keep it parallel to the floor. (Use a full-length mirror to be sure.)

3. Breathe normally while you read the result. Don't cheat by putting extra tension on the tape! Anything more than 35 inches (40 inches for men) is serious cause for concern, according to guidelines from the National Institutes of Health in Bethesda, MD. "That's the level at which your risk of diabetes, high blood pressure, and heart disease rises considerably," explains Dr. Kuczmarski.

2. Learn to graze. Many dieters develop the unfortunate habit of skipping meals, getting most of the day's calories from just one or two large ones, one of which is usually in the evening. That's trouble—especially if you're diabetic, because you need to keep your blood sugar levels steady. Studies have shown that people who spread their food intake over the course of the day take in fewer calories overall and tend to eat more nutritious foods (presumably because their snack choices aren't driven by hunger). The best plan: Eat five or six small meals throughout the day. This will benefit both your waistline and your blood sugar.

3. Take a daily walk. No matter how much you change your diet, abdominal fat isn't going anywhere unless you get up and move. Specifically, it requires aerobic exercise. "As you decrease overall body fat, you'll end up with a leaner waistline," says Kathryn M. Rexrode, MD, associate physician and instructor in the division of internal medicine at Harvard Medical School. Walking is among the best forms of exercise to keep belly fat in check. Dr. Kahn's study found that women who walked regularly were 16% less likely to gain inches at the waist than those who didn't. "There's a major, consistent effect from walking, but you need to walk 4 hours a week, or at least 30 minutes every day, to see it," he says.

4. Tone your tummy. Thin may sound good, but when it comes to abs, toned is what you really want. "Thin people can end up with Pillsbury Doughboy tummies if they don't train their ab muscles specifically," says Len Kravitz, PhD, researcher and exercise scientist at the University of New Mexico in Albuquerque. "Even though they're thin, they're flabby." Our diabetes-busting, ab-strengthening exercise program (below) is the key to getting a belly worth baring. Strong ab muscles also help protect your back.

5. Strength train. "Resistance training is an important component of a belly-slimming workout, because it increases muscle mass throughout the body, helping to boost metabolism," says Dr. Kravitz. The more muscle you develop, whether in your arms, shoulders, back, or wherever, the greater your ability to burn calories before your body can turn them into fat. And building upper body muscles, such as in your arms and shoulders, can make your waistline look smaller! For a complete strength training workout, see chapter 15: "Boost Your Metabolism to Burn More Fat."

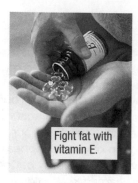

Fight fat with vitamin E.

6. Take vitamin E. There is preliminary evidence that vitamin E may be a potential fat fighter. "It may help prevent abdominal weight gain by protecting against insulin resistance," says Dr. Kahn. And that protection is a big bonus for those with diabetes. Aim for 100 to 400 IU a day. Check with your doctor before taking vitamin E supplements.

7. Stay calm. Crank up the Mozart, take a walk, get a massage, talk to a friend, breathe deeply—do anything that relaxes you. Studies have shown that women who don't control stress tend to have larger waistlines. The culprit appears to be cortisol, a hormone released by the body during periods of stress. It's believed that increased

Three Belly-Busting Moves

Here are three belly-busting moves from Len Kravitz, PhD, of the University of New Mexico in Albuquerque. Do one to three sets of 8 to 12 repetitions each, two or three times a week.

Trunk curls. The everyday crunch is the best. Lie on your back, feet flat on the floor and fingertips lightly supporting your head (or arms folded across your chest). Using your abs, slowly lift your head, shoulders, and upper back off the floor. Hold for a count of two, then lower slowly, and repeat.

Twisting crunches. "Adding a twist to the basic crunch helps target the oblique muscles that run diagonally along your sides," says Dr. Kravitz. Strong obliques are as critical to a tight midsection as strong abs. Start in the same position as above. As you come off the floor, twist your torso, bringing your left shoulder toward your right knee. Be careful not to pull on your neck. Hold for a count of two, then lower slowly. Repeat, alternating sides.

Side bends. This crunch variation helps strengthen the muscles of the entire abdominal area. Start in the same position, and come up as if you're doing a crunch. Keeping your upper body off the floor, bend sideways at the waist, bringing your right elbow toward your right hip. Return to center, then slowly bend sideways to the left. Return to center, lower, and repeat.

TAKE CONTROL: Chart Your Progress

Using an old belt, mark off your current notch with a permanent marker. Hang the belt in your closet or near your bathroom scale. Measure yourself against the belt once a week—and watch the old mark slowly slip away.

cortisol levels play a role in directing fat to the abdominal area.

8. Be social. Having a workout buddy is a great way to help stick to your fitness regimen. And some experts suggest that buddies—even those you don't work out with—can help tone your abs. Those people who reported the most social support from a spouse, family, and friends were the least likely to gain weight during a 3-year study. Researchers say that a wide social network may help reduce stress,

improve self-esteem, and encourage better health practices.

9. Curb the cocktails. Dr. Kahn's study also found that women who drank beer or liquor one to four times a week were more likely to put on abdominal inches than women who didn't imbibe. If you do drink, stick to wine, which was not associated with waist gain and may offer heart-protective effects that beer and liquor may not. Check with your doctor before you drink anything to make sure you're allowed to have alcohol.

CHAPTER 15

Boost Your Metabolism to Burn More Fat

Turn up the calorie burn, and lose more weight by building muscle

Believe it or not, there's a way to lose weight even faster than you would by eating a healthy diet and getting only aerobic exercise. By adding a few simple strength training exercises to your routine, you can burn up to 200 extra calories a day.

How does lifting weights burn so many calories? By building more muscle, you boost your metabolism. And by giving your metabolism an extra boost, you burn more

calories throughout the day—and not just when you're working out. When your metabolism is revved up from a weight workout, you'll burn extra calories even when you're just sitting and watching TV or sleeping! Read on to learn more about how to use metabolism to your weight loss advantage.

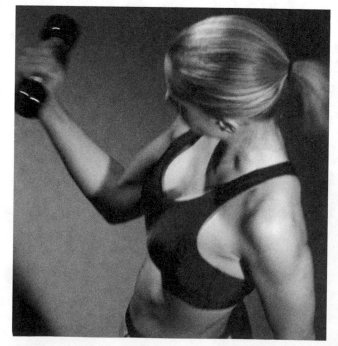

‖ Metabolism 101

Metabolism is all the work your body does that requires calories (energy): staying alive, thinking, breathing, and moving your muscles. Obviously, it plays a major role in how much you weigh, especially with each passing birthday.

Sometime in your 30s, your metabolism starts slowing down by about 5% every decade. That means if you eat about 1,800 calories a day and fit into size 10s when you're 35, you'll be shopping for 12s when you're 45, even if you're eating the same number of calories. By the time you're 55, well, you get the idea.

The culprit behind this decline in calorie-burning is muscle loss, says Steve Farrell, PhD, associate director of The Cooper Institute in Dallas. Every pound of muscle you lose can decrease the number of calories you burn by as many as 30 a day. During perimenopause, you start losing about ½ lb of muscle a year, a loss that can double once you hit menopause. (Blame it on lack of activity and just plain aging.) If you're not careful, by the time you're 65 it's possible to have lost half of your muscle mass and see your metabolism slowed by 200 to 300 calories.

‖ Easy Metabolism Boosters

In addition to weight training (which we'll tell you about next), there are some easy ways to rev up your metabolism.

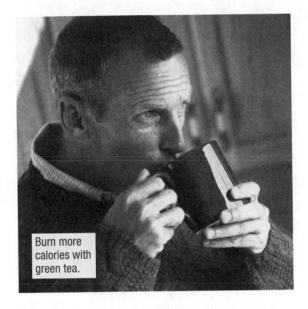

Burn more calories with green tea.

Sip green tea. In a study from Switzerland, 6 out of 10 men who took a green tea supplement three times a day with their meals (the equivalent of a cup of green tea) burned about 80 more calories during the following 24 hours than those who took a caffeine pill or a dummy pill. The researchers believe that flavonoids in the tea were responsible for the metabolism boost.

Savor spicy food. A few small studies from Japan have shown that eating a meal spiced with fiery red pepper may boost metabolism by up to 30%. The downside if you don't love hot food: They used a lot of red pepper—between 5 and 6 teaspoons per meal.

If you work your major muscle groups twice a week, you can expect to replace 5 to 10 years' worth of muscle loss in just a few months.

Lifting weights can literally reverse the aging process, so you look and feel years—maybe even decades—younger.

Have a cup of java. The amount of caffeine (about 135 mg) in an 8-oz cup of brewed coffee is enough to raise your metabolism for more than 2 hours. Drinking it before a workout may give you an extra kick. And caffeine may help free stored fat, so your body can burn it for energy as you exercise. (If you have high blood pressure, avoid caffeine before exercise.)

‖ Rev It Up!

To keep your metabolism chugging in high gear all the time, you need strength training. If you work your major muscle groups twice a week, you can expect to replace 5 to 10 years' worth of muscle loss in just a few months. Lifting weights

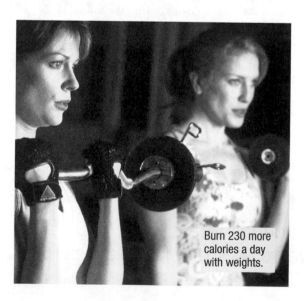

Burn 230 more calories a day with weights.

can literally reverse the aging process, so you look and feel years—maybe even decades—younger.

Lifting weights increases your calorie burn in other ways too. In one study, 15 sedentary people in their 60s and 70s who strength trained 3 days a week for 6 months increased their daily calorie burn by more than 230 calories. Almost one-third of the increase was from a boost in their metabolism due to the muscle they had gained. The remaining calories were burned as a result of their workouts, their increased daily activity, and something called "afterburn," which is an added attraction of strength training exercise. Depending on how hard you work out, explains study author Gary R. Hunter, PhD, of the University of Alabama at Birmingham, your metabolism can stay elevated for up to 48 hours after you've finished lifting.

"As a bonus, strength training builds bone," says Dr. Farrell. "Though we tend to think of bones as 'dead,' they are very alive and highly active. Strong bones use more nutrients, and ultimately they burn more calories than weak bones do."

QUICK TIP: Compete with a Buddy

Even if you and your friend can't work out at the same time, you can still have fun by creating some competition between you. Get together for a workout, and record how much each of you can lift for various exercises. Then do it again in about a month or two to find out which one of you improved the most. Wager $20, a video, or anything else that will motivate you.

A Weight Training/Aerobics Combo Helped Him Lose Big

Doctor's orders made Johnny L. Scott take control of his diabetes. The result? He lost 33 lb and avoided insulin injections. Here's his story.

"At age 24, I weighed 139 lb, but within the next couple of years I was up to 175. Next thing I knew, I was 208. It had to be the sweets; I love sweets. Once I hit 208, my weight stayed steady. I knew my cholesterol was high, and I was eating some fried foods and steak. But I didn't worry about it, because basically I was doing the right things, such as exercising.

"I had to take a physical in December of 1999 so I could renew my Department of Transportation license, just in case UPS needed me to pinch-hit as a driver during the holidays. When the nurse at the clinic told me that my urine test results showed I was diabetic, I was shocked. Nobody in my family had diabetes, and I didn't have any symptoms. I ended up passing the physical for the UPS test, so I convinced myself I wasn't diabetic. But by early February 2000, I was constantly thirsty and constantly going to the bathroom. Whenever I had a lot of sweets, I would get a tremendous headache. After a few of those, I said okay, maybe I'd better go to a doctor to get checked. A blood test showed that I had type 2 diabetes.

"After I was diagnosed, I started exercising religiously—and smarter. I devised a workout program that gives me weight training as well as cardiovascular exercise. I couldn't believe how my body changed after I started running and really eating right. It was a huge change: In 6 months I dropped to 175 and cut my waist size from 34 to 29. I've had all my suits altered. But the best part is that I can control my blood sugar without giving myself insulin shots."

Johnny's Workout

➤ Performs 100 sit-ups in the morning and another 100 at bedtime.

➤ Strength trains 2 days in a row, alternating between pulling exercises (rows, curls) the first day and pushing exercises (bench presses, dips) the next; rests a day; then works out the next 2 days by doing the same push and pull routines.

➤ Runs about 1 mile each workout day.

‖ The Workout

Because these exercises challenge more than one muscle group at a time, you'll build calorie-burning muscle fast. Here's how they work: Do 10 to 12 repetitions of each exercise, then rest for 30 to 60 seconds between exercises. Do this workout three times a week, allowing a day of rest in between. For best results, use an amount of weight that will be difficult to lift during your last few reps.

SQUAT: From a standing position, with legs shoulder-width apart, bend at the knees and hips, and lower yourself as though you're sitting down. Keep your back straight, and make sure you can always see your toes. Stop just shy of touching the chair, then stand back up. For more of a challenge, hold a dumbbell in each hand.

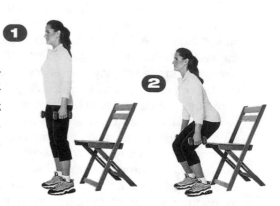

LUNGE: Standing with your feet together, step back about 2 to 3 feet with your right foot. Bending your left knee, slowly lower yourself. Keep your left knee directly over your ankle. Before your right knee touches the floor, push off with your right foot, and return to the starting position. Repeat with your left leg.

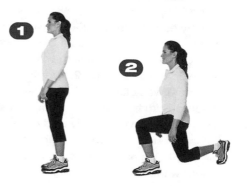

LAT PULL-DOWN: In a seated position, hold an exercise band above your head with your arms almost straight and your hands about shoulder-width apart. The band should be taut, but not pulled tight. Bending your left arm, pull your elbow down toward your hip. Slowly release. Repeat with your right arm.

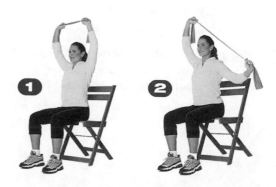

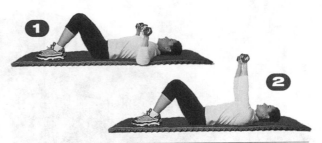

CHEST PRESS: Lying on your back, hold dumbbells just above chest height with your elbows pointing out. Slowly press the dumbbells straight up, extending your arms. Slowly lower.

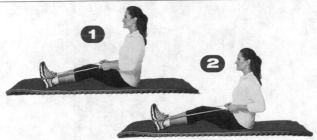

SEATED ROW: In a seated position with your arms extended in front of you, hold an exercise band so it's taut, but not pulled tight. Squeeze your shoulder blades together, and pull your hands back toward your rib cage. Your elbows should be close to your body and pointing back. Slowly release.

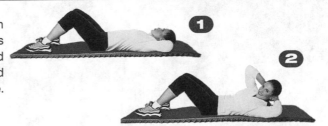

DIAGONAL CURL-UP: Start by lying down with your feet flat on the floor, legs bent, and knees pointed toward the ceiling. Slowly lift your head and shoulders off the floor, twist to the left, and bring your right shoulder toward your left knee. Slowly lower. Repeat, alternating sides.

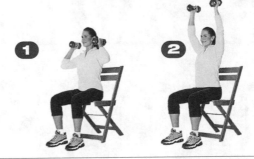

OVERHEAD PRESS: While seated, hold dumbbells at shoulder height, palms facing in. Press the dumbbells straight overhead, then slowly lower.

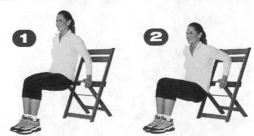

CHAIR DIP: Keeping your shoulders down and your back straight, bend your elbows back, and lower your butt toward the floor as far as comfortably possible. Slowly push back up.

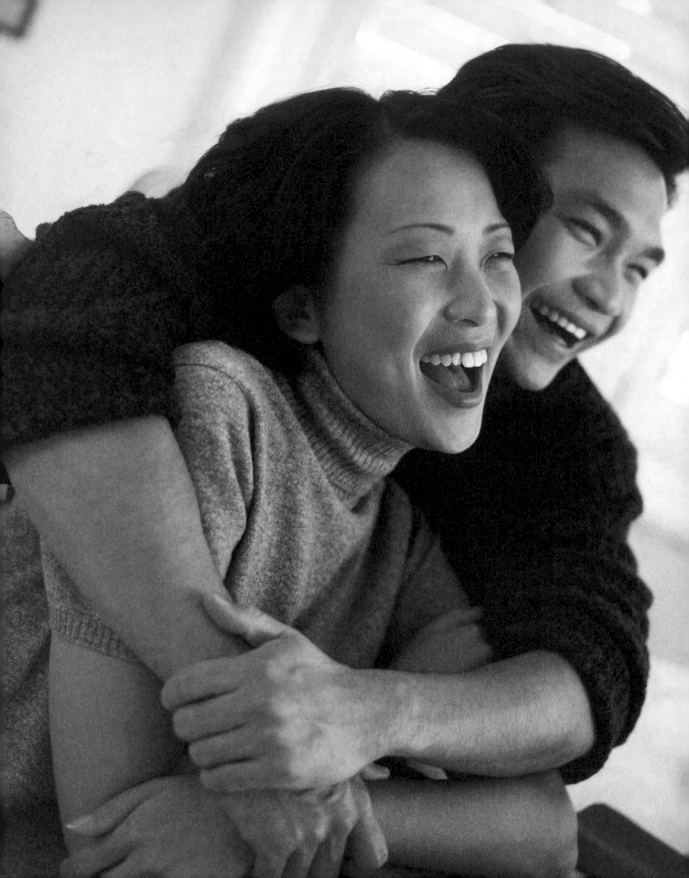

PART FIVE

Prevent Diabetes Complications

Keep both minor and major side effects at bay with the right preventive care

CHAPTER 16

Stay Healthy from Head to Toe

Avoid diabetes-related complications by taking some simple preventive measures

Whether you're newly diagnosed with diabetes or have had the disease for years, your doctor has probably made you aware of other health problems that diabetes can bring about—from an increased risk of gum disease and foot problems all the way to heart disease.

But don't worry—there are some basic measures you can take that will decrease your chances of experiencing such complications. These preventive steps are as simple as getting yearly checkups, taking good care of your skin, and watching your blood sugar levels (something you're already doing). In addition to following a healthy diet and exercise regimen (like the ones outlined in this book), practice the health tips presented in this chapter and you'll be looking forward to a long and healthy life!

Vision Problems

Statistics say that the overwhelming majority of diabetics—90% to be exact—who have had the condition for 15 years or longer will notice vision problems and changes to the eyes. Though clues arc few, experts believe that the small blood vessels that supply the retina with vital oxygen and nutrients are damaged by the decrease in circulation due to diabetes. In turn, damaged blood vessels lead to damage in the thin, light-sensitive tissue that lines the back of the eye and sends images through the optic nerve to the brain. People with diabetes are almost twice as likely to develop glaucoma. In glaucoma, pressure builds up in the eye, causing irreparable damage to the retina and optic nerve.

But don't get discouraged. There are things you can do to protect your vision so you're less likely to have these problems.

Keep your blood sugar and blood pressure stable. You can help prevent eye problems simply by monitoring your glucose levels and having your blood pressure checked regularly.

Get a yearly eye exam. Schedule an annual trip to the eye doctor. Damage occurs long before you notice a change in your vision (such as blurriness, eye pain, or double vision), so this is the best way to keep problems from getting serious, explains Marian Parrott, MD, vice president of clinical affairs at the American Diabetes Association (ADA). Pregnancy can worsen diabetic eye disease, so plan to get a comprehensive eye exam before you become pregnant, and see your ophthalmologist during the first trimester. She'll be able to tell you if you need to be followed more closely while you're expecting.

If your diabetes has already led to eye problems, your doctor can offer a variety of laser treatments to seal leaky capillaries and prescribe medication to help prevent vision-related symptoms.

Gum Disease

Diabetes puts you at greater risk for gum disease, for two reasons. First, diabetes decreases the amount of saliva in your mouth—saliva that would normally help wash away plaque. Second, because people with diabetes tend to have higher blood sugar levels in their saliva, the growth of plaque and germs is increased. Blood sugar in your saliva is no better for your teeth than sugar in your coffee.

Advanced stages of diabetes can cause problems with nerves and blood vessels in the mouth. Loss of collagen, the tissue that supports skin, gums, and bone, along with decreased circulation, puts your teeth at greater risk of periodontal disease. To keep teeth and gums in top form, brush up on these tips.

See a pro. You should of course brush your teeth at least twice daily and floss at least once, but it's also very important to visit your dentist every

---

TAKE CONTROL: Have a Healthy Smile

Another reason to see the dentist at least every 6 months: Just as diabetes can lead to dental complications, oral disease can aggravate blood sugar problems. In fact, dental infections can make it tougher for you to keep your blood sugar levels stable. So if you haven't seen the dentist recently, make an appointment today.

For a healthy smile, brush up on dental hygiene and keep blood sugar in check.

3 to 6 months. He can monitor your gum health and offer special antibacterial plaque treatments to protect your gums.

Watch blood sugar levels. Controlling glucose levels in your bloodstream will help relieve existing oral infections and gum disease as well as prevent future problems. In fact, keeping blood sugar stable can help strengthen the cells that defend us from all kinds of infections, explains Enrique Caballero, MD, of the Joslin Diabetes Center in Boston.

‖ Skin Woes

Because of decreased bloodflow and increased blood sugar, people with diabetes may experience a greater incidence of rashes, inflammation, local-ized itching, or other skin problems. And poorly controlled blood sugar can interfere with the healing of even minor abrasions. Here's how to make sure your skin stays healthy and heals the way it should.

Administer first-aid fast. To prevent infections, cleanse cuts and scrapes with gentle soap and water as soon as you notice them. Then, if your doctor approves, apply antibiotic cream. Avoid harsh antiseptic treatments, especially those that contain alcohol.

Guard against irritation and dryness. When showering or bathing, use mild and unscented soaps, and avoid feminine hygiene sprays. Keep skin moisturized, especially in cold, dry weather.

See a professional. Consult a dermatologist if you can't solve a skin problem yourself. And see your physician if you have recurring yeast infections or if a course of over-the-counter treatment fails to rid you of this problem. Recurrent yeast infections indicate poor diabetes control (yeast thrive on high blood sugar).

A Better Skin Balm

A spray-on skin balm derived from a human gene—the first drug to emerge from the Human Genome Project, an effort to map the human genetic code—helped chronic venous ulcers heal more completely in people with circulatory problems. These ulcers are common among people with diabetes. Current treatments can take months and are often unsuccessful.

In a study performed by Human Genome Sciences, a private research lab based in Rockville, MD, 63 people used repifermin twice a week for up to 12 weeks. Repifermin is a spray-on balm made of a protein called keratinocyte growth factor-2 (KGF-2). Participants had skin ulcers for as long as 3 years before entering the study. They saw a significant acceleration in partial wound healing compared with those who did not use the drug, says researcher David C. Stump, MD.

‖ Foot Problems

People who experience tingling or numbness in their feet as a result of diabetes need to pay particular attention to foot care, because these symptoms indicate decreased circulation and nerve damage. When nerves aren't working properly in the feet, you may not notice if you get injured there, which can lead to problems such as infection. Reduced bloodflow can also make foot injuries take longer to heal. Here are ways to make sure your feet stay healthy.

Practice daily care. Wash your feet daily in warm water, and dry them well, especially between the toes. Apply skin lotion or petroleum jelly on the tops and bottoms of your feet (but not between the toes) to keep them from drying and cracking. Use talcum powder between the toes to prevent fungus.

Put them in motion. Promote circulation to your feet by taking regular walks and stretching your toes and ankles periodically throughout the day.

Be protective. Wear nice, warm socks in extreme cold, and apply sunscreen to feet when they'll be exposed to sun. Most important of all: Never walk barefoot. Invest in comfortable, well-fitting shoes. Before putting them on, always check inside and remove any debris that could rub you the wrong way. Get rid of shoes made of plastic or vinyl and ones that chafe or otherwise irritate your feet.

Heal Foot Ulcers Faster

The next time you get a foot ulcer—a common problem for those with diabetes—you may want to ask your doctor about a new treatment: a bioengineered "skin" recently approved by the FDA that could help the ulcer heal faster.

The skin, called Apligraf, is made from donated human skin cells. In a study of 33 foot ulcer patients, those who got standard ulcer care and had their ulcers dressed with the skin healed about twice as quickly as those who got standard care alone, according to Aristidis Veves, MD, who headed the study and is the research director of the microcirculation lab at Joslin Beth Israel Deaconess Foot Center in Boston.

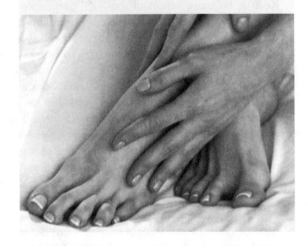

TAKE CONTROL: Take Your Toes to a Pro

If you have difficulty keeping your balance when clipping your toenails, you may want to consider paying a podiatrist to cut them for you. In more advanced stages, diabetes can lead to dizziness and eye problems that can make toe clipping more difficult.

Give them the once-over. Do a daily foot check for trouble spots such as blisters or cuts, and treat them immediately. (See "Administer first-aid fast" on p. 94.) If you have a wound that seems to be taking a long time to heal, call your doctor to discuss treatment options.

See a podiatrist yearly. Schedule a complete foot exam annually. If you notice a tingling or numbness in your feet (or hands), tell your doctor right away. These symptoms may signal nerve damage in these areas.

‖ Bladder Infections

Bladder infections can be common in people who have had diabetes for a while, since nerve-related side effects of the disease may make it difficult for you to feel when your bladder is full. It can also be tough to tell when you've emptied your bladder completely. Here's what you can do to keep this organ healthy.

Don't "hold it." Schedule bathroom breaks once every 2 to 3 hours, even if you don't feel you have to go. Dr. Parrot also suggests taking

---

Double Trouble: Diabetes Plus Hypertension

If you have diabetes and high blood pressure, the National Kidney Foundation (NKF) has a special message—and a new treatment—for you. "People with these two conditions are at increased risk for cardiovascular problems as well as kidney disease," says William Keane, MD, president of the NKF and professor of medicine at the University of Minnesota Medical School in Minneapolis. "The key is to keep even closer control of blood pressure than experts have recommended in the past." If you're one of the 11 million Americans with both conditions, make a doctor's appointment today, and discuss the points listed below. "Despite the severity of these medical problems, people are largely unaware of the dangers," Dr. Keane says. "The following recommendations give doctors the tools that will save lives."

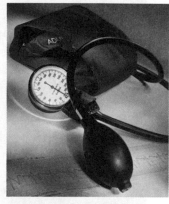

Aim for these numbers. If you're diabetic, work with your physician to achieve a blood pressure less than 130/80. Check it monthly until you've reached this goal, Dr. Keane suggests.

Discuss meds with your doctor. The NKF recommends aggressive treatment that could involve several medications, including ACE inhibitors that help prevent blood vessel contraction, diuretics that help rid the body of excess water waste, long-acting calcium channel blockers that relax blood vessels, and beta-blockers that slow heart rate. The good news: Early treatment may forestall the need for more meds in the future.

Take action at home. While lifestyle changes haven't proved as potent at fighting off the repercussions of hypertensive diabetes, they are still worth pursuing, says Dr. Keane. Minimize fat, cholesterol, and salt in your diet, and don't smoke.

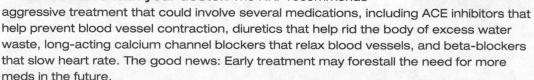

the direct approach: "If you have a bladder that doesn't contract very well, press down on your abdomen to make sure your bladder is completely empty," she advises.

Control blood sugar levels. "Glucose is a good venue for growing bacteria," notes Robert Sherwin, MD, past president of the ADA and director of the Diabetes Endocrinology Research Center at Yale University. That means that bacteria can thrive in urine left in the bladder for long periods of time. This can lead to an infection that could, if left untreated, affect the kidneys too. By keeping your blood sugar under control, you'll remove the "food" for these bacteria.

Know when to see the doctor. Make an appointment if you're having incontinence problems or suspect that you have a bladder infection (which may require antibiotic treatment). If you're experiencing lower-back pain, it may be a sign of a severe kidney infection. Your physician can give you a simple test to make sure your kidneys are functioning properly.

‖ Heart Disease

To keep blood flowing freely, you've got to keep your blood sugar levels in check. But it doesn't hurt to keep your blood levels of cholesterol and fat to a minimum either. This is especially important with diabetes, because this condition puts

Pay Attention to Postmeal Blood Sugar Spikes

Diabetics normally monitor their fasting blood sugar levels, but a study from the Finnish government found that testing blood sugar 2 hours after a meal is a more accurate predictor of heart disease risk. "Spikes in blood sugar levels show up after meals. If these spikes go untreated, they can increase a patient's risk for future illness," says Robert Gabbay, MD, PhD, director of the diabetes program at Pennsylvania State University in State College. If postmeal glucose levels are higher than 180, talk to your doctor. Prescription drugs, including Glyset, Precose, and Prandin, can lower elevated levels.

you at greater risk for heart disease. Keep your heart healthy with these tips.

Say no to naughty foods. Experts agree that you should keep the salt and fat in your diet to a minimum. If you have high blood pressure and need to reduce your sodium intake, eat more fresh foods and fewer processed ones, or at least read labels so you'll know how much sodium you're getting. Make sure you get no more than 2,400 mg sodium per day. Focus on lowering your

TAKE CONTROL: Kick the Habit

If you're a smoker, you're aggravating nearly all the complications that people with diabetes already face, especially those related to bloodflow. "The combination of diabetes and smoking gives you two different factors that affect your circulation," says Enrique Caballero, MD, of the Joslin Diabetes Center in Boston. Fortunately, once you quit—regardless of how long you've been a smoker—your health will improve. And the quitting regimen is the same for people with diabetes as for everyone else, which means it's okay to use special aids such as nicotine patches and gum.

TAKE CONTROL: Avoid Wacky Diets

Experts recommend that you don't try any odd eating trends such as the high-protein diets that recently gained popularity. Such unbalanced diets may put undue strain on your body. Instead, stick to a well-rounded, low-fat, high-fiber diet.

fat intake to no more than 60 g a day and eating more fruits and vegetables. See chapter 6 for a complete healthy eating plan based on the Diabetes Food Exchange System.

Get in the exercise habit. Get moving to further strengthen your circulatory system. Easy exercise such as walking will help *all* of your body's organs function their best and lower your blood sugar naturally.

Inquire about aspirin. Aspirin relieves pain, but it also helps prevent the blood clotting that can block circulation. Many physicians now recommend that their diabetic patients take one aspirin every day. Ask your doctor if you should.

‖ Impotence

Unfortunately, diabetes can lead to impotence if it damages large and small arteries and nerve pathways that affect the penis or other parts of the abdomen. Between 35 and 50% of men with diabetes experience impotence, but you can keep your reproductive system functioning properly by following this advice.

Have a plan. Seek a physician's guidance to help keep your blood pressure down, your glucose levels even, and your diet low in salt—all of which will help keep your sexual organs in good working order.

Seek diagnosis and treatment. There can be many causes of impotence besides diabetes. Only a doctor can pinpoint the actual cause, which will determine the necessary treatment. Drugs such as Viagra work for people with diabetes, though you might require a stress test or some cardiac testing before your doctor will prescribe this medication.

CHAPTER 17

Get Relief from Nerve Pain

Ease this painful side effect with the latest treatments and best self-care advice

O ne of the unfortunate side effects some people with diabetes may experience is a condition called diabetic neuropathy. It happens when high blood sugar levels damage nerve endings, which carry signals between the brain or spinal cord and the muscles, skin, and internal organs. The result of this damage is stabbing, tingling, and burning sensations in the legs, hands, and feet, especially at night.

Fortunately, researchers are finding effective new ways to treat this painful condition. They've discovered that a special dietary supplement and a side effect–free prescription drug both can help to quell the nerve pain, making it possible for you to lead a more pain-free life. Keep reading to find out how these discoveries, along with good self-care habits, can help you to feel better.

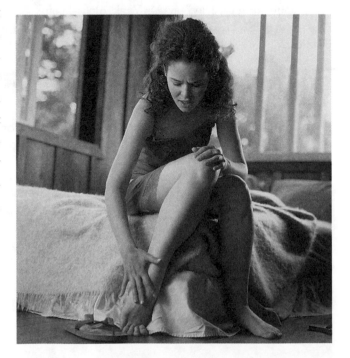

Antioxidant Treats Neuropathy Symptoms

It's been called "nature's best-kept secret." Alpha-lipoic acid—a little-known compound produced by your body—is a superantioxidant, maybe even more powerful than vitamins C and E and beta-carotene. Studies prove that alpha-lipoic acid prevents free radical damage to your cells, in part by recycling vitamins C and E. But where it shows real promise is in relieving diabetic neuropathy. "Preliminary studies in Europe have been very promising," says Aaron Vinik, MD, PhD, director of the Strelitz Diabetes Research Institute at the Eastern Virginia Medical School in Norfolk.

In fact, alpha-lipoic acid works so well that in Germany it is a prescription drug for diabetic neuropathy. "There is a lot of new evidence that diabetic neuropathy is caused in part by oxidative stress, and that people with diabetes have deficient antioxidant capacity," says Dr. Vinik. Alpha-lipoic acid may replenish that deficiency. A 4-year clin-

Good Self-Care

If you suffer from peripheral neuropathy, try these helpful pain-easing tips.
➤ If your feet burn, use a capsaicin cream to quell the pain.
➤ Inspect your feet twice a day for wounds and punctures.
➤ Wear comfy shoes when you walk.
➤ Carefully navigate your walking terrain (in advance, if possible) to avoid falls.

ical trial began last year at several centers in the US and Europe to answer whether alpha-lipoic acid is an effective treatment of the underlying neuropathy. Alpha-lipoic acid may also help control blood sugar levels in diabetics. One German study found that 600 mg alpha-lipoic acid a day improved blood sugar regulation in people with type 2 diabetes.

Early evidence for using alpha-lipoic acid to treat diabetic neuropathy and regulate blood sugar is convincing. Dr. Vinik estimates that as many as

Alpha-Lipoic Acid at a Glance

Name: Alpha-lipoic (pronounced Al-fa-ly-PO-ic) acid

Benefit: Acts as a powerful antioxidant. At doses of 600 to 1,200 mg a day, it may relieve the pain of diabetic neuropathy and help control blood sugar levels.

Cost: Some examples we found: Nature's Way alpha-lipoic acid, 60 capsules of 50 mg each, $14.59 ($2.92 a day for 600 mg); and Natrol alpha-lipoic acid, 50 capsules of 300 mg each, $29.25 ($1.17 a day for 600 mg)

Cautions: Only minor side effects such as headache and nausea have been reported, even at high doses.

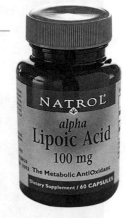

TAKE CONTROL: Get a Second Opinion

If you suspect that you have peripheral neuropathy and think you've been misdiagnosed, don't hesitate to get a second opinion. Many doctors aren't aware of the condition and thus miss it.

15% of endocrinologists in the US now prescribe it to their patients with diabetes. But there's no use trying to get enough alpha-lipoic acid from your diet: Foods have tiny amounts of the antioxidant. For example, it takes 7 lb of spinach to produce just 1 mg alpha-lipoic acid. That's a lot of spinach!

If you're going to try it: In the studies that have been conducted, only large doses of alpha-lipoic acid have proven helpful. Opt for two to four 300-mg capsules a day. If you choose lower-strength capsules, you might have to take as many as 24 a day to reach an effective dose. And, as with any supplement, be sure to let your doctor know what you are taking.

Drug Helps Pain without Side Effects

One medication eases the searing pain of diabetic neuropathy—and improves sleep—without the sedation, confusion, or bowel problems other commonly prescribed medications can cause, according to research from the Southwestern Vermont Medical Center in Bennington. The study of 135 people found that those who took the prescription drug gabapentin (Neurontin) had greater pain control in just 2 weeks and better sleep in 1 week, says Keith Edwards, MD, director of clinical research at the facility's Neurological Research Center.

Learn More about Neuropathy

The Neuropathy Association offers educational materials, referrals to neurologists, and help finding (or starting) a support group. The nonprofit group's mission—further advanced with each $25 member donation—is to support research to find a cure for this disease. For more information, call (800) 247-6968. You can also write to them at 60 E. 42nd St., Suite 942, New York, NY 10165-0999. Or visit their Web site at www.neuropathy.org.

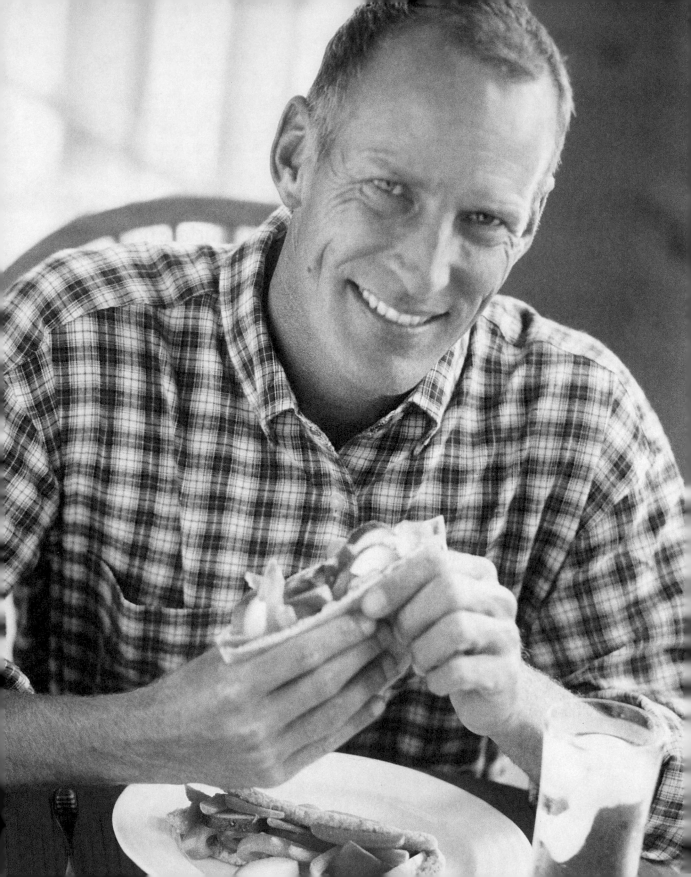

PART SIX

70 Delicious Healing Recipes

*Enjoy great-tasting meals, snacks, and even desserts
that are healthy for both you and your family*

All the Flavor—And Good for You Too!

Enjoy all the tastes and foods you love—and still control your diabetes

It used to be that having diabetes meant being forced to adopt a diet of only bland, tasteless food. That's because the things that make food taste great—such as generous amounts of fat and sugar—are off-limits to diabetics.

But times have changed. Now we know of other ways to cook up great flavor and still keep recipes low in fat, cholesterol, sugar, and sodium. To show you just how well you can eat when you have diabetes, we've created a collection of 70 delectable dishes that are also perfectly healthy. And the diet exchanges for each recipe are included, making it easy to keep track of your food intake for the day.

Get ready to enjoy!

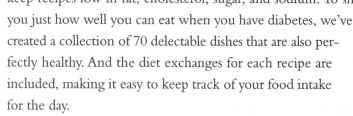

CHAPTER 18

Breakfast

Start your day off with one of these eight delicious breakfasts that will help keep your blood sugar under control

‖ Fruit and Nut Granola Cereal

Always a great source of fiber, granola is typically coated in oil or butter before baking, making it high in fat. We substituted frozen apple juice concentrate for most of the oil.

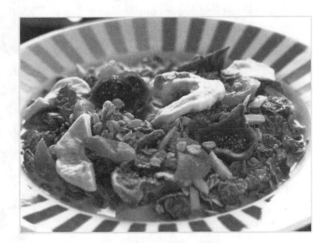

2	**c rolled oats**
1	**c wheat flakes**
2	**Tbsp sunflower seeds**
1½	**Tbsp sesame seeds**
¼	**c frozen apple juice concentrate, thawed**
¼	**c packed brown sugar**
2	**Tbsp canola oil**
½	**tsp ground cinnamon**

¼	**c chopped dried figs**
¼	**c chopped dried apple rings**
¼	**c chopped dried apricots**
¼	**c slivered toasted almonds**

1. Preheat the oven to 250°F. Coat a jelly-roll pan with cooking spray.
2. In a medium bowl, combine the oats, wheat flakes, seeds, apple juice concentrate, sugar, oil, and cinnamon. Toss to mix well.
3. Spread the oat mixture in the prepared pan. Bake, stirring occasionally, for 45 minutes, or until golden brown. Let cool slightly.
4. Stir in the figs, apples, apricots, and almonds. Store in an air-tight container in a cool, dry place for up to 2 weeks.

Makes 10 ⅔-cup servings

Per serving: 212 cal, 5 g pro, 35 g carb, 7 g fat, 1 g sat. fat, 0 mg chol, 5 g fiber, 8 mg sodium
Diet exchanges: 0 milk, 0 vegetable, 1 fruit, 1½ bread, 0 meat, 1 fat

Jumbo Cinnamon-Raisin Muffins

Whole grain pastry flour and low-fat yogurt increase the fiber and reduce the fat in these muffins.

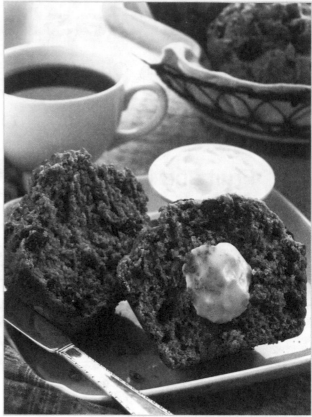

2	c whole grain pastry flour
½	c packed brown sugar
2	tsp baking powder
1	tsp ground cinnamon
½	tsp salt
¼	tsp baking soda
¾	c raisins
2	lg egg whites
1	c low-fat plain or vanilla yogurt
1	Tbsp maple syrup
1	tsp vanilla extract

1. Preheat the oven to 350°F. Coat a 6-cup jumbo muffin pan with cooking spray.
2. In a medium bowl, combine the flour, sugar, baking powder, cinnamon, salt, and baking soda. Stir in the raisins.
3. In a small bowl, beat the egg whites lightly. Stir in the yogurt, maple syrup, and vanilla extract. Stir into the flour mixture just until combined. Evenly divide the batter among the prepared cups.
4. Bake for 35 minutes, or until a wooden pick inserted into the center of a muffin comes out clean. Cool on a rack for 5 minutes. Remove the muffins from the pan, and cool completely.

Makes 6 muffins

Per muffin: 322 cal, 9 g pro, 72 g carb, 1 g fat, 0 g sat. fat, 0 mg chol, 6 g fiber, 440 mg sodium
Diet exchanges: 0 milk, 0 vegetable, 1 fruit, 3 bread, 0 meat, 0 fat

Apple-Walnut Muffins

Chopped fresh apples and whole grain pastry flour add fiber while low-fat buttermilk is substituted for some of the oil in these hearty muffins.

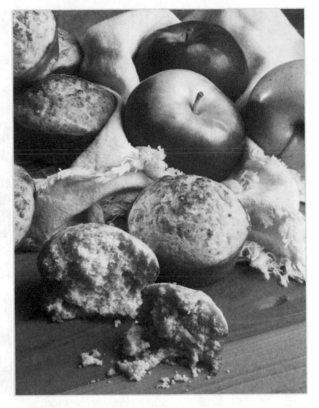

1½	**c whole grain pastry flour**
2	**tsp baking powder**
1	**tsp baking soda**
½	**tsp ground cinnamon**
¼	**tsp salt**
½	**c low-fat buttermilk**
3	**Tbsp vegetable oil**
¼	**c packed brown sugar**
1	**egg**
½	**c finely chopped, peeled apples**
½	**c golden raisins (optional)**

1. Preheat the oven to 400°F. Coat a 12-cup muffin pan with cooking spray.
2. In a medium bowl, combine the flour, baking powder, baking soda, cinnamon, and salt.
3. In a large bowl, combine the buttermilk, oil, sugar, and egg. Stir in the flour mixture just until combined. Stir in the apples and raisins, if using.
4. Evenly divide the batter among the prepared cups. Bake for 13 minutes, or until a wooden pick inserted in the center of a muffin comes out clean. Cool on a rack for 5 minutes. Remove the muffins from the pan, and cool completely.

Makes 12 muffins

Per muffin: 116 cal, 3 g pro, 18 g carb, 4 g fat, 0 g sat. fat, 18 mg chol, 2 g fiber, 238 mg sodium
Diet exchanges: 0 milk, 0 vegetable, 0 fruit, 1 bread, 0 meat, 1 fat

‖ Fluted Egg Cups

Reduced-fat cheese eliminates the saturated fat content of this dish. Always use whole wheat or whole grain bread to get the most fiber.

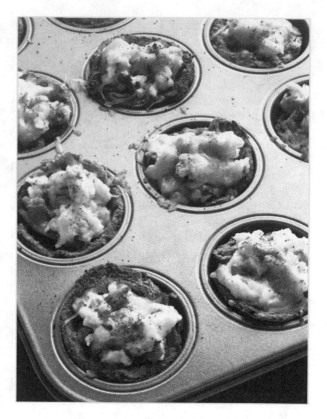

6	slices whole wheat bread
1	tsp olive oil
⅓	c chopped scallions
1	Tbsp chopped fresh basil
1	Tbsp chopped fresh Italian parsley
8	egg whites, lightly beaten
	Salt and ground black pepper
⅓	c reduced-fat shredded Cheddar cheese
1	Tbsp grated Parmesan cheese

1. Preheat the oven to 350°F.
2. With a rolling pin, slightly flatten the bread slices. Using a 3"-round cookie cutter, cut 12 bread circles. Coat a 12-cup mini-muffin pan with cooking spray, and line each cup with a bread round. Bake for 15 minutes, or until the edges are golden. Preheat the broiler.
3. Heat the oil in a nonstick skillet over medium heat, and cook the scallions, basil, and parsley for 2 minutes. Add the egg whites. Season with salt and pepper. Cook, stirring, for 2 minutes, or until almost set. Add the Cheddar, and cook until the cheese has melted and the eggs are set.
4. Evenly divide the egg mixture among the bread cups, and sprinkle with the Parmesan. Broil 4 inches from the heat for 1 minute, or until hot and golden.

Makes 6 servings

Per serving: 116 cal, 10 g pro, 14 g carb, 2 g fat, 0 g sat. fat, 2 mg chol, 2 g fiber, 208 mg sodium
Diet exchanges: 0 milk, 0 vegetable, 0 fruit, 1 bread, 1 meat, 0 fat

Garden Bounty Omelettes

Using two egg whites and one whole egg per omelette reduces the fat and cholesterol. The tomatoes and pepper add fiber and antioxidants.

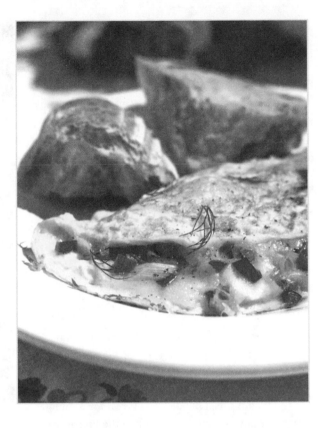

3	**plum tomatoes, chopped**
1	**red bell pepper, chopped**
2	**scallions, chopped**
¼	**c chopped fresh dill**
4	**egg whites**
2	**eggs**
2	**tsp fat-free milk**
	Salt and ground black pepper
4	**Tbsp shredded reduced-fat smoked Jarlsberg cheese**

1. Heat a medium nonstick skillet coated with cooking spray over medium heat. Cook the tomatoes, red pepper, scallions, and dill for 7 minutes, or until soft. Place in a small bowl.
2. Wipe out the skillet, and coat with cooking spray. Return to the heat.
3. In a medium bowl, whisk the egg whites, eggs, and milk. Season with salt and pepper. Pour half of the egg mixture into the skillet, and cook, occasionally scraping the bottom of the pan, for 3 minutes. Sprinkle half of the vegetable mixture over the eggs, and top with 2 tablespoons of the cheese. Continue to cook for 3 to 4 minutes, or until the cheese is melted, the bottom is golden brown, and the eggs are set.
4. Using a large spatula, flip the omelette in half, and place on a plate. Keep warm.
5. Repeat to make another omelette.

Makes 2 servings

Per serving: 179 cal, 19 g pro, 10 g carb, 7 g fat, 2 g sat. fat, 218 mg chol, 2 g fiber, 306 mg sodium
Diet exchanges: 0 milk, 1½ vegetable, 0 fruit, 0 bread, 2½ meat, 1 fat

Great Western Quiche

Low-fat Canadian bacon gives a smoky flavor, and evaporated milk offers a rich substitute for high-fat half-and-half.

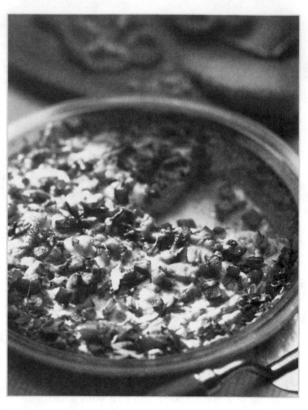

1	**bunch scallions, sliced**
1	**sm green bell pepper, chopped**
2	**oz Canadian bacon, chopped**
½	**c shredded reduced-fat Cheddar cheese**
1	**c fat-free evaporated milk**
¾	**c liquid egg substitute**
2	**tsp Dijon mustard**
¼	**tsp ground nutmeg**
1	**Tbsp grated Parmesan cheese**

1. Preheat the oven to 350°F. Coat a pie pan with cooking spray.
2. Heat a medium nonstick skillet coated with cooking spray over medium heat. Cook the scallions, bell pepper, and bacon for 3 minutes, or until softened. Spoon into the prepared pie pan. Top with the Cheddar.
3. In a large bowl, combine the milk, egg substitute, mustard, and nutmeg. Pour into the pie pan. Sprinkle with the Parmesan.
4. Bake for 35 minutes, or until golden and a knife inserted in the center comes out clean.

Makes 6 servings

Per serving: 108 cal, 12 g pro, 8 g carb, 3 g fat, 1 g sat. fat, 11 mg chol, 1 g fiber, 367 mg sodium
Diet exchanges: ½ milk, ½ vegetable, 0 fruit, 0 bread, 1 meat, ½ fat

‖ Rich Vanilla Waffles

Fat-free yogurt moistens these waffles, reducing the need for added butter—and also making the waffles a source of calcium. Top with fresh fruit for fiber-rich sweetness.

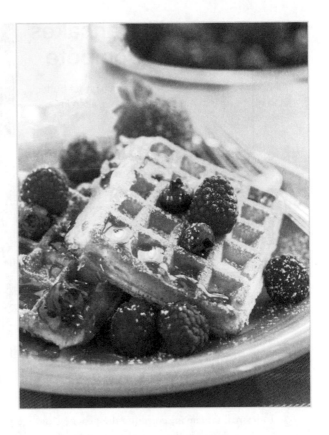

¾	**c fat-free milk**
¾	**c fat-free vanilla yogurt**
2	**egg yolks**
1	**Tbsp canola oil**
¾	**c cake flour**
2	**tsp baking powder**
½	**tsp baking soda**
¼	**tsp salt**
½	**c sugar**
4	**egg whites**

1. Preheat a waffle iron according to the manufacturer's directions.
2. In a small bowl, combine the milk, yogurt, egg yolks, and oil.
3. In a large bowl, combine the flour, baking powder, baking soda, salt, and ¼ cup of the sugar. Stir in the milk mixture.
4. Place the egg whites in a medium bowl. Using an electric mixer, beat on medium speed until foamy. Gradually beat in the remaining ¼ cup sugar on high speed until soft peaks form. Fold the egg white mixture into the batter.
5. Spoon a scant ¾ cup batter into the center of the waffle iron. Cook until the waffle is golden brown and crispy. (Do not press on the iron during cooking, or the waffle will collapse.) Repeat to make a total of 10 waffles.

Makes 10 servings

Per serving: 180 cal, 5 g pro, 33 g carb, 2 g fat, 1 g sat. fat, 43 mg chol, 0 g fiber, 246 mg sodium
Diet exchanges: 0 milk, 0 vegetable, 0 fruit, 2 bread, 0 meat, ½ fat

Buttermilk Pancakes with Fruit Compote

Change your pancake topping from high-fat butter and high-sugar syrup to fiber-packed, vitamin- and mineral-rich fruit.

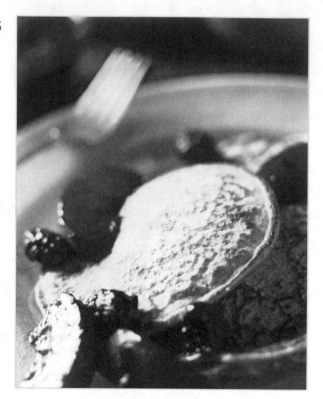

2	peaches or nectarines, sliced
¼	c orange juice
3	Tbsp apricot preserves
¼	tsp ground cinnamon
1	c blackberries
2	c whole grain pastry flour
1	Tbsp sugar
1	tsp baking soda
½	tsp baking powder
½	tsp salt
1	egg
1	egg white
2	c low-fat buttermilk
1	Tbsp vanilla extract
2	tsp canola oil

1. In a small saucepan, combine the peaches, orange juice, preserves, and cinnamon. Cook over medium heat for 5 minutes, or until the fruit is soft. Add the blackberries, and cook for 2 minutes. Keep warm over very low heat.
2. In a large bowl, combine the flour, sugar, baking soda, baking powder, and salt.
3. In a medium bowl, whisk the egg and egg white until very foamy. Whisk in the buttermilk, vanilla extract, and oil. Stir into the flour mixture just until combined.
4. Heat a large nonstick skillet coated with cooking spray over medium heat. Pour ⅓ cup batter into the skillet to form a 4" pancake. Repeat to fit as many pancakes in the skillet as possible. Cook for 3 minutes, or until bubbles appear on the surface. Turn, and cook for 2 minutes, or until golden brown. Transfer to a warm oven.
5. Repeat to make a total of 12 pancakes. Serve the pancakes with the warm compote.

Makes 12 servings

Per serving: 139 cal, 5 g pro, 26 g carb, 2 g fat, 0 g sat. fat, 19 mg chol, 4 g fiber, 274 mg sodium
Diet exchanges: 0 milk, 0 vegetable, ½ fruit, 1½ bread, 0 meat, 0 fat

CHAPTER 19

Lunch

Whip up a quick soup, salad, or sandwich from this collection of 10 healing recipes

‖ Pasta e Fagiole

The white beans in this dish are a great source of fiber, and research links fiber-rich diets to less diabetes and other chronic diseases.

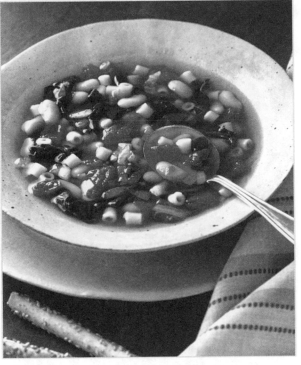

2	tsp olive oil
1	sm onion, chopped
2	cloves garlic, chopped
2	cans (14½ oz each) fat-free chicken broth
1	can (15 oz) diced tomatoes
1	can (15 oz) cannellini or white beans, rinsed and drained
½	c ditalini or other small pasta
½	lb Swiss chard or spinach leaves, coarsely chopped

1. Heat the oil in a Dutch oven over medium heat. Cook the onion and garlic, stirring occasionally, for 3 minutes, or until soft.
2. Add the broth, tomatoes, beans, and pasta. Cook, stirring, for 15 minutes, or until the pasta is cooked. Add the Swiss chard and cook, stirring, for 2 minutes, or until the chard is wilted.

Makes 6 servings

Per serving: 127 cal, 9 g pro, 21 g carb, 2 g fat, 0 g sat. fat, 0 mg chol, 5 g fiber, 479 mg sodium
Diet exchanges: 0 milk, 1 vegetable, 0 fruit, 1 bread, ½ meat, ½ fat

Mushroom-Barley Soup

Soaking dried vegetables such as mushrooms or tomatoes in boiling water creates a very quick, flavorful broth that's sodium-free. You can also use dried veggies with store-bought broth to reduce the sodium in soups and stews.

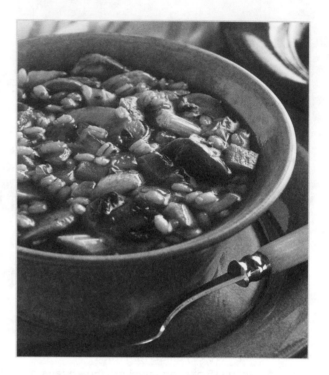

1	oz dried morel or porcini mushrooms
3	c boiling water
1	lg onion, chopped
2	carrots, chopped
1	rib celery, chopped
12	oz cremini or button mushrooms, stems removed, sliced
1½	tsp dried oregano
2	cans (14½ oz each) fat-free chicken broth
½	c barley

1. Place the dried mushrooms in a small bowl. Cover with the boiling water, and let stand.
2. Meanwhile, coat a large saucepan with cooking spray. Add the onion, carrots, and celery. Coat lightly with cooking spray. Cook over medium heat, stirring often, for 3 minutes. Add the sliced mushrooms and oregano. Cook, stirring, for 7 minutes, or until all the vegetables are soft. Add the broth and barley, and cook for 15 minutes.
3. Line a mesh sieve with a coffee filter or paper towel. Strain the dried mushroom water into the saucepan. Remove and discard the filter or paper towel. Rinse the dried mushrooms under running water to remove any grit. Chop, and add to the saucepan.
4. Cook for 15 minutes, or until the barley is tender.

Makes 6 servings

Per serving: 131 cal, 9 g pro, 25 g carb, 0 g fat, 0 g sat. fat, 0 mg chol, 5 g fiber, 131 mg sodium
Diet exchanges: 0 milk, 2 vegetable, 0 fruit, 1 bread, ½ meat, 0 fat

Balsamic-Lentil Soup

Adding chopped escarole (or spinach or any other dark green leaf) to soups and stews is a great way to increase your intake of vegetables while also adding nice flavor to the dish.

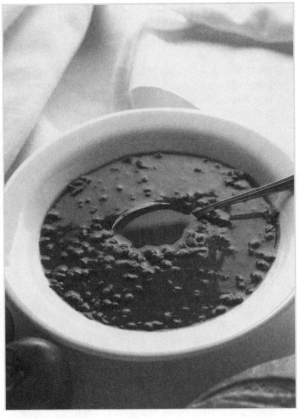

2	tsp olive oil
1	onion, chopped
2	cloves garlic, minced
3	c vegetable broth
3	c water
1	can (14½ oz) diced tomatoes
1	c dried lentils, sorted and rinsed
2	c chopped escarole
2	Tbsp balsamic vinegar

1. Heat the oil in a large saucepan over medium-high heat. Add the onion, and cook, stirring, for 5 minutes, or until soft. Add the garlic, and cook for 1 minute.
2. Add the broth, water, tomatoes, and lentils. Bring to a boil. Reduce the heat to low, cover, and simmer for 40 minutes, or until the lentils are tender.
3. Stir in the escarole and vinegar. Cook for 5 minutes to blend the flavors.

Makes 4 servings

Per serving: 226 cal, 5 g pro, 38 g carb, 4 g fat, 0 g sat. fat, 0 mg chol, 13 g fiber, 897 mg sodium
Diet exchanges: 0 milk, 2 vegetable, 0 fruit, 2 bread, ½ meat, ½ fat

Santa Fe Stuffed Sandwiches

Canned beans replace high-fat, high-sodium cold cuts in this tasty sandwich. Rinsing canned beans reduces their sodium content by one-third.

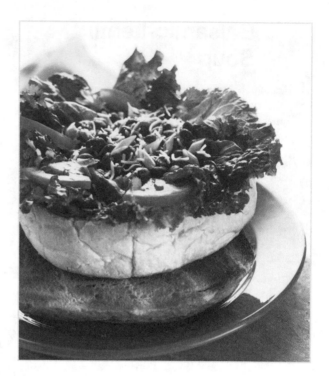

1	unsliced round (12 oz) multigrain or sourdough bread
1	can (19 oz) black beans, rinsed and drained
2	scallions, sliced
2	Tbsp chopped fresh cilantro or parsley
¼	c spicy barbecue sauce
5	lg leaves lettuce
1	c shredded low-fat Monterey Jack cheese
1	tomato, thinly sliced
2	roasted red peppers

1. With a serrated knife, slice off the top third of the bread. Set aside. Hollow out the bottom, leaving a ½"-thick shell. Reserve the bread pieces for another use.

2. In a medium bowl, coarsely mash half the beans. Stir in the scallions, cilantro, barbecue sauce, and the remaining beans.

3. Line the hollowed bread with the lettuce. Cover with the bean mixture. Top with the cheese, tomato, and peppers. Cover with the reserved bread top, and press firmly. Cut into 6 wedges.

Makes 6 servings

Per serving: 303 cal, 16 g pro, 46 g carb, 6 g fat, 3 g sat. fat, 14 mg chol, 7 g fiber, 896 mg sodium
Diet exchanges: 0 milk, 1 vegetable, 0 fruit, 2½ bread, 1 meat, ½ fat

Grilled Cheese Sandwiches

Spraying the bread slices with cooking spray gives these sandwiches the crispiness of butter without the fat and calories.

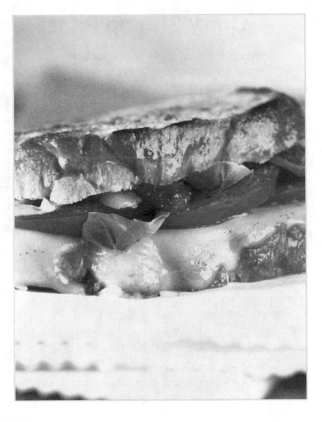

8	**slices (8 oz) semolina or sourdough bread, sliced diagonally**
8	**slices (1 oz each) low-fat Jarlsberg cheese**
1	**lg tomato, cut into 8 slices**
2	**roasted red peppers, halved**
12	**lg leaves fresh basil**

1. Coat both sides of the bread with olive oil cooking spray. In a large nonstick skillet, cook the bread on one side over medium heat for 2 minutes, or until lightly toasted. Do this in batches, if necessary. Remove from the skillet.
2. Arrange 4 of the slices, toasted side up, on a work surface. Top each with 2 slices of cheese, 2 slices of tomato, 1 slice of pepper, and basil. Top with the remaining bread slices, toasted sided down.
3. Place the 4 sandwiches in the skillet. Cook for 2 minutes per side, or until toasted and the cheese melts.

Makes 4 servings

Per serving: 253 cal, 13 g pro, 36 g carb, 6 g fat, 3 g sat. fat, 16 mg chol, 3 g fiber, 480 mg sodium
Diet exchanges: 0 milk, 1 vegetable, 0 fruit, 2 bread, 1 meat, ½ fat

‖ Curry Shrimp Pitas

Adding chopped fruit to these sandwiches
increases the fiber, and the almonds provide
some healthy monounsaturated fat.

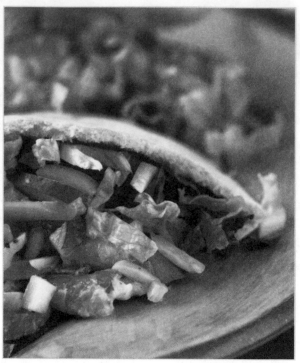

½	**c low-fat mayonnaise**
¼	**c hot mango chutney**
1	**Tbsp soy sauce**
1	**Tbsp curry powder**
¾	**lb cold cooked and peeled shrimp**
2	**ribs celery, chopped**
2	**nectarines, chopped**
¼	**c slivered almonds, toasted**
6	**whole wheat pitas**
2	**c shredded romaine lettuce**

1. In a large bowl, combine the mayonnaise,
   chutney, soy sauce, and curry powder.
   Add the shrimp, celery, nectarines, and
   almonds. Toss to coat.
2. Cut each pita in half crosswise. Evenly divide
   the lettuce and shrimp salad among the pita halves.

Makes 6 servings

Per serving: 353 cal, 17 g pro, 49 g carb, 11 g fat, 2 g sat. fat, 88 mg chol, 7 g fiber, 767 mg sodium
Diet exchanges: 0 milk, 1 vegetable, ½ fruit, 2½ bread, 1½ meat, 1½ fat

Mexican Cobb Salad

Turkey bacon and fat-free cheese keep the fat and calories down in this south-of-the-border salad. In addition, avocado and buttermilk create a creamy dressing that's packed with nutritious monounsaturated fat.

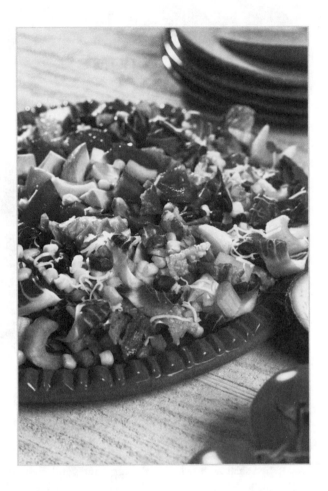

1	lg head romaine lettuce, chopped
1	package (10 oz) frozen corn kernels, thawed
1	can (15 oz) black beans, rinsed and drained
1	lg tomato, chopped
2	ribs celery, chopped
1	green bell pepper, chopped
1	red onion, chopped
1½	c shredded fat-free Monterey Jack cheese
8	slices turkey bacon, cooked and crumbled
1	ripe avocado, cut into chunks
1½	c low-fat buttermilk
2	Tbsp lime juice
½	tsp hot-pepper sauce

1. Arrange the lettuce on a large platter. Arrange the corn, beans, tomato, celery, bell pepper, onion, cheese, and bacon crosswise in strips over the lettuce.
2. In a food processor or blender, combine the avocado, buttermilk, lime juice, and hot-pepper sauce. Process until smooth. Drizzle over the salad.

Makes 8 servings

Per serving: 223 cal, 16 g pro, 26 g carb, 7 g fat, 2 g sat. fat, 16 mg chol, 7 g fiber, 574 mg sodium
Diet exchanges: 0 milk, 1½ vegetable, 0 fruit, 1 bread, 1½ meat, 1 fat

Sesame Chicken Fingers

Oven-frying the chicken eliminates the excess oil of deep-frying. Oven-frying also works well with pork or veal cutlets or chops.

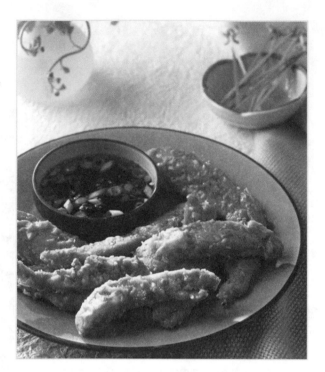

⅔	c soy sauce
6	Tbsp rice wine vinegar
7	Tbsp water
3	scallions, sliced
2½	Tbsp sugar
1	Tbsp grated fresh ginger
1½	tsp toasted sesame oil
½	tsp crushed red-pepper flakes
1½	lb boneless, skinless chicken breasts, cut into ¾"-wide strips
2	egg whites
¾	c whole grain pastry flour
3	Tbsp sesame seeds, toasted

1. In a medium bowl, combine the soy sauce, vinegar, 6 tablespoons of the water, scallions, sugar, ginger, oil, and red-pepper flakes. Transfer ⅓ cup of the sauce to a large bowl. Cover and refrigerate the remaining sauce.
2. Add the chicken to the sauce in the large bowl. Toss well to coat. Let marinate for 15 minutes.
3. In a shallow bowl, beat the egg whites and the remaining 1 tablespoon of the water. In another shallow bowl, combine the flour and sesame seeds.
4. Preheat the oven to 350°F. Coat a baking sheet with cooking spray.
5. Dip the chicken strips into the egg white mixture and then into the flour mixture, shaking off any excess. Place on the baking sheet. Coat the chicken with cooking spray. Bake for 5 minutes. Remove from the oven, and turn the chicken strips. Coat with cooking spray. Bake for 5 minutes longer, or until golden and cooked through.
6. Serve with the sauce on the side.

Makes 10 servings

Per serving: 165 cal, 19 g pro, 11 g carb, 2 g fat, 0 g sat. fat, 39 mg chol, 2 g fiber, 793 mg sodium
Diet exchanges: 0 milk, 0 vegetable, 0 fruit, ½ bread, 2½ meat, ½ fat

Mediterranean Chickpea Salad

Use extra virgin olive oil in salads. It imparts a lot of flavor—even when you use just a small amount of it.

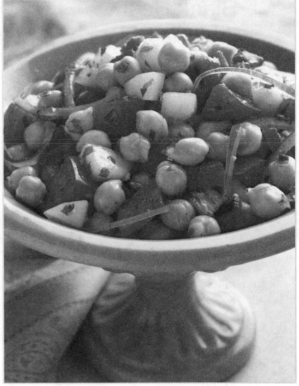

1	**can (15 oz) chickpeas, rinsed and drained**
3	**plum tomatoes, chopped**
1	**roasted red pepper, chopped**
½	**sm red onion, quartered and thinly sliced**
½	**cucumber, peeled, halved, seeded, and chopped**
2	**Tbsp chopped fresh oregano or 1 tsp dried**
2	**cloves garlic, minced**
3	**Tbsp lemon juice**
2	**tsp extra virgin olive oil**
¼	**tsp salt**

In a large bowl, combine all the ingredients, tossing to coat well. Let stand for 10 minutes for the flavors to blend.

Makes 4 servings

Per serving: 154 cal, 6 g pro, 24 g carb, 6 g fat, 0 g sat. fat, 0 mg chol, 8 g fiber, 320 mg sodium
Diet exchanges: 0 milk, 1 vegetable, 0 fruit, 1 bread, 0 meat, 1 fat

Black Bean Jicama Salad

Jicama, the Mexican potato, is a brown-skinned vegetable ranging in size from an orange to a football. To prepare, just peel the skin and cut into slices. It has the texture of a water chestnut and is slightly sweet and low in calories.

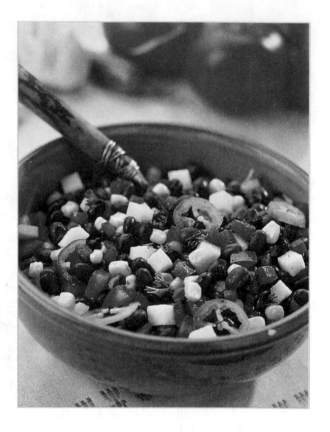

3	c cooked black beans (from scratch; or canned, rinsed, and drained)
2	tomatoes, chopped
1	c chopped jicama
2	red bell peppers, finely chopped
1	c yellow corn (off the cob or frozen thawed)
3	jalapeño chile peppers, chopped (for a slightly less hot taste, remove the seeds)
3	cloves garlic, minced
2	Tbsp chopped fresh cilantro
1	Tbsp cumin
1	Tbsp olive oil
3	Tbsp lime juice
1	Tbsp red wine vinegar
	Salt and ground black pepper to taste

In a large salad bowl, combine all the ingredients. Cover, and refrigerate for at least 2 hours.

Makes 8 servings

From The Diabetes Food & Nutrition Bible: A Complete Guide to Planning, Shopping, Cooking, and Eating *by Hope Warshaw, MMSc, RD, CDE, and Robyn Webb, MS (American Diabetes Association, 2001; $18.95/trade paperback)*

Per serving: 146 cal, 7 g pro, 27 g carb, 2 g fat, 0 g sat. fat, 0 mg chol, 8 g fiber, 90 mg sodium
Diet exchanges: 0 milk, 1 vegetable, 0 fruit, 2½ bread, 0 meat, 0 fat

CHAPTER 20

Dinner

Choose from 27 delicious dinners that will satisfy your tastebuds *and* take care of your body

‖ Macaroni and Cheese

Changing the pasta in your recipes to the whole wheat variety increases the fiber content and also adds a nutty flavor.

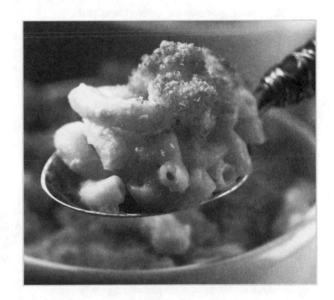

½	**lb whole wheat elbow macaroni**
¼	**c all-purpose flour**
½	**tsp dry mustard**
2½	**c 1% milk**
1½	**c shredded reduced-fat extra-sharp Cheddar cheese**
2	**Tbsp dry bread crumbs**
2	**Tbsp grated Parmesan cheese**

1. Preheat the oven to 350°F. Coat a 2½-quart baking dish with cooking spray.
2. Prepare the macaroni per package directions.
3. Place the flour and mustard in a medium saucepan. Gradually add the milk, whisking constantly, until smooth. Place over medium heat. Cook, whisking constantly, for 8 minutes, or until thickened. Remove from the heat. Stir in the cheese until smooth. Stir in the macaroni, and place in the prepared baking dish.
4. Sprinkle the bread crumbs and Parmesan over the macaroni. Bake for 20 minutes, or until heated through.

Makes 6 servings

‖ **Per serving:** 306 cal, 18 g pro, 40 g carb, 8 g fat, 4 g sat. fat, 28 mg chol, 1 g fiber, 315 mg sodium
‖ **Diet exchanges:** ½ milk, 0 vegetable, 0 fruit, 2½ bread, 1 meat, 1 fat

‖ Eggplant Parmesan

Avoid the extra calories and fat of frying by oven-frying eggplant. The breaded slices are coated with cooking spray before baking to create a crispy, browned crust.

2	**med eggplants, peeled and cut crosswise into ¼"-thick slices**
2	**eggs**
2	**egg whites**
1½	**c seasoned dry bread crumbs**
1	**jar (26 oz) pasta sauce**
2	**c shredded low-fat mozzarella cheese**
⅓	**c grated Parmesan cheese**

1. Preheat the oven to 450°F. Coat two baking sheets and a 13" x 9" baking dish with cooking spray.
2. Place the eggplant in a single layer on the prepared baking sheets. Bake for 15 minutes, or until soft.
3. Meanwhile, beat the eggs and egg whites in a shallow bowl. Place the bread crumbs in another bowl. Dip the eggplant slices into the egg mixture and then into the bread crumbs, pressing to coat. Place on the baking sheets. Coat with cooking spray.
4. Bake the eggplant for 5 minutes, or until golden. Turn the slices. Coat with the spray, and bake for 5 minutes longer, or until golden.
5. Lower the oven temperature to 350°F. Spread one-third of the pasta sauce in the prepared baking dish. Top with half of the eggplant slices, half of the mozzarella, and half of the Parmesan. Spread one-third of the pasta sauce over the cheese. Top with the remaining eggplant slices. Spread the remaining one-third pasta sauce, and sprinkle with the remaining cheese. Bake for 30 minutes, or until heated through.

Makes 8 servings

‖ **Per serving:** 283 cal, 16 g pro, 32 g carb, 10 g fat, 5 g sat. fat, 73 mg chol, 5 g fiber, 973 mg sodium
Diet exchanges: 0 milk, 3 vegetable, 0 fruit, 1 bread, 1½ meat, 1 fat

‖ Baked Ziti

Eating protein with pasta helps keep blood sugar balanced. In this dish, chicken provides not only protein but also great flavor—and with less fat than beef.

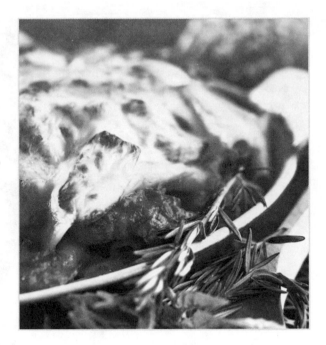

½   lb whole wheat ziti
½   lb boneless, skinless chicken breasts, cut into thin strips
1   lg onion, chopped
¼   c chopped sun-dried tomatoes (dry pack)
2   cloves garlic, minced
2   Tbsp balsamic vinegar
1   can (28 oz) tomatoes in thick puree
2   tsp Italian seasoning
1   c shredded reduced-fat mozzarella cheese

1. Preheat the oven to 350°F. Coat a 2½-quart baking dish with cooking spray.
2. Prepare the ziti per package directions. Place in a large bowl.
3. Heat a large skillet coated with cooking spray over medium heat. Add the chicken, and cook, stirring, for 5 minutes, or until browned. Remove to a bowl. Recoat the skillet, and cook the onion and sun-dried tomatoes for 5 minutes, or until soft. Add the garlic, and cook for 2 minutes. Add the vinegar, and cook for 2 minutes, stirring to loosen any brown bits. Stir in the canned tomatoes (with puree), Italian seasoning, and chicken. Simmer for 15 minutes. Add to the bowl with the ziti, and toss.
4. Place half of the ziti mixture in the prepared dish. Sprinkle with half of the cheese. Top with the remaining ziti mixture and the remaining cheese. Bake for 25 minutes, or until heated through.

Makes 4 servings

Per serving: 370 cal, 30 g pro, 52 g carb, 6 g fat, 3 g sat. fat, 49 mg chol, 7 g fiber, 541 mg sodium
Diet exchanges: 0 milk, 3 vegetable, 0 fruit, 2 bread, 3 meat, ½ fat

‖ Chicken Potpie

No need to skip rich potpie—this healthy version has a creamy broth made with low-fat milk. The potpie is then topped with low-fat biscuits for a tasty "crust."

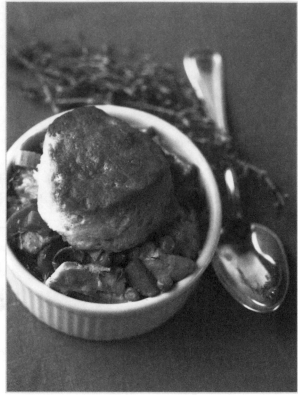

1	tsp olive oil
1	lg onion, chopped
8	oz button mushrooms, sliced
1	tsp dried thyme
½	c fat-free chicken broth
⅓	c all-purpose flour
1	c 1% milk
2	c cooked chicken breasts (½ lb), cut into 1" cubes
2	c frozen peas and carrots
	Salt and ground black pepper
1	tube (7½ oz) low-fat biscuit dough

1. Preheat the oven to 425°F. Coat a 9" x 9" baking dish with cooking spray.
2. Heat the oil in a large saucepan over medium heat. Add the onion, mushrooms, and thyme, and cook, stirring often, for 8 minutes, or until the vegetables are tender. Add the broth, and cook for 2 minutes, stirring to loosen any brown bits.
3. Place the flour in a small bowl. Whisk in the milk until smooth. Add to the saucepan along with the chicken and peas and carrots. Cook, stirring constantly, over medium heat for 6 minutes, or until the mixture thickens and begins to bubble. Season with salt and pepper.
4. Place the mixture in the prepared baking dish. Top with the biscuits. Bake for 10 minutes, or until the biscuits are golden brown and cooked through.

Makes 4 servings

Per serving: 403 cal, 31 g pro, 57 g carb, 7 g fat, 2 g sat. fat, 47 mg chol, 7 g fiber, 913 mg sodium
Diet exchanges: ½ milk, 3½ vegetable, 0 fruit, 2½ bread, 2½ meat, ½ fat

Quick Chicken Gumbo

Broth-based soups and stews that are loaded with vegetables make a healthy, satisfying meal. You can pump up the veggies in this recipe by adding some of your family's favorites.

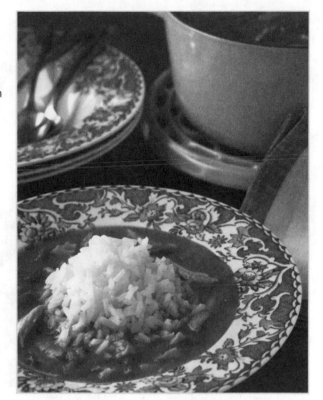

⅓	**c white or brown rice**
2	**tsp olive oil**
1	**sm onion, chopped**
1	**sm green bell pepper, chopped**
2	**ribs celery, chopped**
2	**cloves garlic, chopped**
1	**tsp dried thyme**
2	**cans (14½ oz each) fat-free chicken broth**
2	**c shredded cooked boneless, skinless chicken breasts (½ lb)**
1	**can (8 oz) tomato sauce**
1	**c water**

1. Prepare the rice per package directions.
2. Heat the oil in a Dutch oven over medium heat. Add the onion, pepper, celery, garlic, and thyme, and cook, stirring, for 7 minutes, or until the vegetables are soft.
3. Stir in the broth, chicken, tomato sauce, and water. Cook, stirring occasionally, for 15 minutes to blend the flavors.
4. To serve, spoon the gumbo into shallow bowls. Top each serving with ¼ cup of the rice.

Makes 4 servings

Per serving: 222 cal, 24 g pro, 20 g carb, 4 g fat, 1 g sat. fat, 44 mg chol, 2 g fiber, 469 mg sodium
Diet exchanges: 0 milk, 1½ vegetable, 0 fruit, 1 bread, 3 meat, ½ fat

‖ White Chicken Chili

Chicken substitutes beautifully for fattier beef in this wholesome chili. The baked chips add fiber, flavor, and crunch without extra fat.

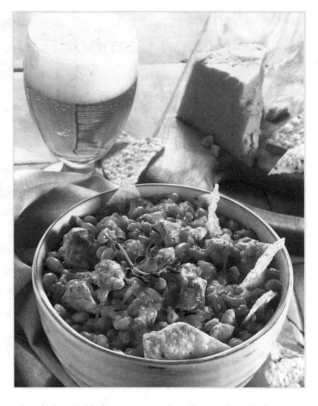

¾	**lb boneless, skinless chicken breast, cubed**
1	**lg onion, chopped**
2	**cloves garlic, minced**
1	**c chicken broth**
2	**cans (12 oz each) navy beans, rinsed and drained**
1	**tsp ground cumin**
½	**tsp salt**
⅛	**tsp ground red pepper**
4	**c baked tortilla chips**
½	**c shredded reduced-fat extra-sharp Cheddar cheese**

1. Heat a large skillet coated with cooking spray over medium-high heat. Add the chicken, and cook for 10 minutes, or until no longer pink, stirring frequently. Remove, and set aside. Recoat the skillet. Add the onion and garlic, and cook for 5 minutes, or until soft.
2. Place the chicken, onion, and garlic in a slow cooker. Add the broth, beans, cumin, salt, and pepper. Simmer on low for 5 to 6 hours. Serve over the tortilla chips, topped with the cheese.

Makes 8 servings

Per serving: 185 cal, 17 g pro, 23 g carb, 4 g fat, 1 g sat. fat, 30 mg chol, 4 g fiber, 678 mg sodium
Diet exchanges: 0 milk, ½ vegetable, 0 fruit, 1½ bread, 1½ meat, ½ fat

Baked Chicken and Vegetable Couscous

High-fat sour cream marinades are made healthier by substituting fat-free yogurt, as we did in this recipe. Using a flavored yogurt, such as lemon, adds zest without extra work.

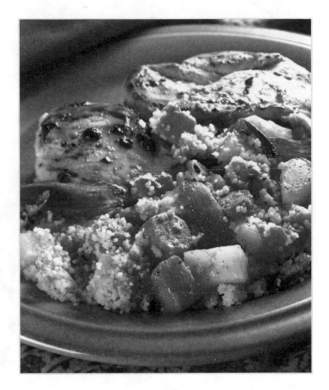

1	c fat-free lemon yogurt
2	cloves garlic, minced
1	Tbsp grated fresh ginger
2	tsp curry powder
4	skinless chicken breast halves
4	carrots, cut into 1" pieces
4	parsnips, cut into 1" pieces
1	sm butternut squash, cut into 1" pieces
1	red onion, cut into 1" pieces
1	Tbsp olive oil
1½	c fat-free chicken broth
½	box (5 oz) whole wheat couscous

1. In a 13" x 9" baking dish, combine the yogurt, garlic, ginger, and curry powder. Add the chicken, turning to coat. Cover, and refrigerate for at least 4 hours or up to 12 hours.
2. When the chicken has marinated, preheat the oven to 400°F. Place the carrots, parsnips, squash, onion, and oil in a large roasting pan. Toss to coat. Bake for 30 minutes, or until tender.
3. Meanwhile, remove the chicken from the refrigerator, and stir in the broth. Cover loosely with foil, and bake along with the vegetables for 25 minutes. Remove both from the oven. Remove the foil from the chicken, and place the vegetables around it. Bake, uncovered, for 15 minutes.
4. Prepare the couscous per package directions. Fluff with a fork, and serve with the chicken and vegetables.

Makes 4 servings

Per serving: 574 cal, 48 g pro, 85 g carb, 6 g fat, 1 g sat. fat, 83 mg chol, 17 g fiber, 254 mg sodium
Diet exchanges: 0 milk, 5 vegetable, 0 fruit, 3 bread, 5 meat, 1 fat

Chicken Stew with Dumplings

Whole grain pastry flour is finely ground and substitutes well for white flour in baked goods such as these dumplings. Because it's not as refined as white flour, whole grain pastry flour contains all the nutrients and fiber of the whole grain.

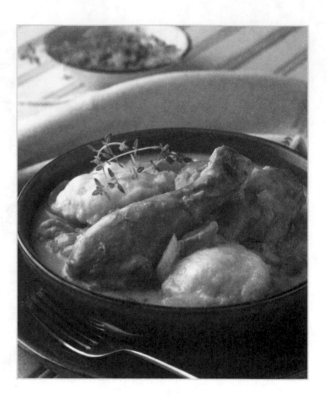

2	lb chicken parts, skinned
	Salt
2	onions, chopped
2	carrots, sliced
2	ribs celery, sliced
3	c fat-free chicken broth
1	tsp dried thyme
½	c low-fat sour cream
2	Tbsp + 1 c whole grain pastry flour
1½	tsp baking powder
½	c buttermilk
1	egg white, lightly beaten

1. Sprinkle the chicken with the salt. Coat lightly on all sides with cooking spray.
2. Cook the chicken in a large pot over medium-high heat for 5 minutes, until browned on all sides. Remove to a plate.
3. Coat the same pot with cooking spray. Add the onions, carrots, and celery, and cook over medium-high heat for 5 minutes, stirring occasionally. Add the broth, thyme, and chicken. Bring to a boil over high heat. Reduce the heat to medium-low, and simmer for 10 minutes.
4. In a small bowl, whisk together the sour cream and 2 tablespoons of the flour. Stir into the chicken mixture until thickened.
5. In a medium bowl, combine the remaining 1 cup flour and the baking powder. Stir in the buttermilk and egg white just until mixed. The batter will be slightly lumpy.
6. Drop the batter by tablespoonfuls onto the chicken mixture. Cover the pot, and simmer for 25 minutes, or until the chicken and dumplings are cooked through.

Makes 4 servings

Per serving: 415 cal, 48 g pro, 43 g carb, 5 g fat, 3 g sat. fat, 95 mg chol, 8 g fiber, 485 mg sodium
Diet exchanges: ½ milk, 2 vegetable, 0 fruit, 1½ bread, 5½ meat, ½ fat

Roast Chicken with Vegetables

Cooking chicken with the skin on keeps the meat moist and tender. Just be sure to discard the skin before eating the chicken to save fat and calories.

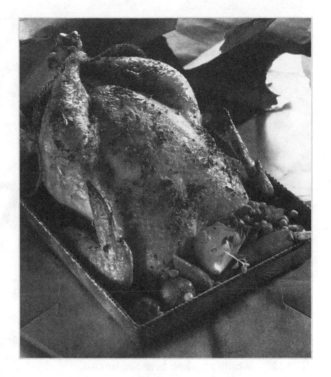

3	cloves garlic, minced
½	tsp salt
½	tsp freshly ground black pepper
1	chicken (about 3½ lb)
1	lb sm red potatoes, quartered
2	carrots, cut diagonally into 1½" pieces
1	onion, cut into wedges
3	Tbsp orange juice concentrate
3	Tbsp red wine vinegar
1	Tbsp olive oil
2	tsp fennel seeds, crushed
½	c frozen peas, thawed

1. Preheat the oven to 375°F. In a small bowl, combine the garlic, salt, and pepper.
2. Rinse the chicken, and pat dry with paper towels. Remove and discard any excess fat. Place the chicken, breast side up, on a rack in a roasting pan. Loosen the skin from the breast meat, and spread the garlic mixture under the skin.
3. In a large bowl, combine the potatoes, carrots, onion, orange juice concentrate, vinegar, oil, and fennel seeds. Arrange the vegetable mixture around the chicken. Roast the chicken, basting occasionally, for 40 minutes. Cover with foil and roast, basting occasionally, for 40 minutes longer, or until a thermometer inserted in a breast registers 180°F and the juices run clear. Add the peas to the pan during the last 10 minutes of roasting.
4. Remove the chicken to a serving platter. Using a slotted spoon, remove the vegetables to the platter with the chicken. Let stand for 10 minutes. Skim the fat from the pan drippings, and discard the fat. Serve the pan juices alongside the chicken and vegetables.
5. Remove the skin from the chicken before eating.

Makes 6 servings

Per serving: 354 cal, 40 g pro, 25 g carb, 11 g fat, 3 g sat. fat, 106 mg chol, 4 g fiber, 337 mg sodium
Diet exchanges: 0 milk, 1 vegetable, 0 fruit, 1 bread, 5 meat, 1½ fat

Grilled Chicken Breasts with Fruit Salsa

Jazz up chicken with this tasty fruit salsa—you'll get great flavor without adding fat.

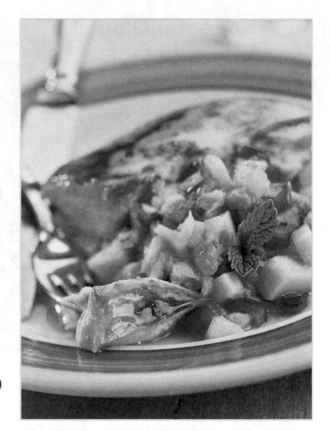

Salsa

2	cans (8 oz each) crushed pineapple, packed in juice, drained
1	mango, peeled and cubed
1	papaya, peeled and cubed
2	Tbsp rice vinegar
1	Tbsp finely chopped cilantro
1	Tbsp chopped red pepper

Chicken

2	whole chicken breasts, boned, skinned, and halved (10 oz meat each)
1	tsp olive oil
	Kiwifruit slices (garnish)

1. In a medium bowl, combine the salsa ingredients. Cover, and refrigerate for 1 hour.

2. Preheat an outdoor grill or oven broiler. Brush the chicken breasts with the oil. Grill or broil the chicken for about 7 minutes per side, or until no pink remains.

3. To serve, place the fruit salsa on a plate, using a few spoonfuls per person. Top with a cooked chicken breast. Garnish with kiwi slices.

Makes 4 servings

From The Diabetes Food & Nutrition Bible: A Complete Guide to Planning, Shopping, Cooking, and Eating *by Hope Warshaw, MMSc, RD, CDE, and Robyn Webb, MS (American Diabetes Association, 2001; $18.95/trade paperback)*

Per serving: 305 cal, 32 g pro, 30 g carb, 6 g fat, 2 g sat. fat, 85 mg chol, 3 g fiber, 79 mg sodium
Diet exchanges: 0 milk, 0 vegetable, 2 fruit, 0 bread, 4 very lean meat, 1 fat

Spicy Pecan-Crusted Trout

Toasting nuts enhances their natural flavor and allows you to use a small enough amount to get their healing benefits without too much fat or too many calories.

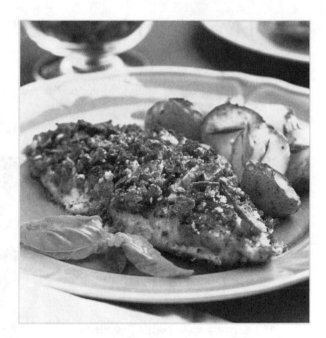

3	scallions, chopped
2	Tbsp reduced-sodium teriyaki sauce
1	clove garlic, minced
4	rainbow trout, cod, or red snapper fillets (6 oz each), skinned
1	c fresh whole wheat bread crumbs
½	c whole grain cereal flakes, coarsely crushed
¼	c toasted pecans, chopped
2	Tbsp shredded fresh basil

1. In a glass baking dish or shallow bowl, combine the scallions, teriyaki sauce, and garlic. Add the fillets, turning to coat both sides. Cover, and refrigerate for 1 to 2 hours.
2. In a pie plate, combine the bread crumbs, cereal, and pecans. Remove the trout from the marinade one at a time, and place in the pie plate. Press into the crumb mixture to coat all sides. Repeat with the remaining fillets, discarding the marinade.
3. Heat a large nonstick skillet coated with cooking spray over medium heat. Add the trout, and cook for 3 minutes, or until browned. Coat the top of the fillets with cooking spray. Turn, and cook for 4 minutes, or until browned and the fish flakes easily when tested with a fork. Sprinkle with the basil.

Makes 4 servings

Per serving: 406 cal, 39 g pro, 15 g carb, 21 g fat, 4 g sat. fat, 100 mg chol, 4 g fiber, 313 mg sodium
Diet exchanges: 0 milk, ½ vegetable, 0 fruit, 1 bread, 5 meat, 3½ fat

‖ Five-Alarm Shrimp

A small serving of a flavorful dish such as this one
will satisfy you better than a large portion of a bland
meal. Garlic, chile pepper, citrus juice, and herbs
add the zing to this spicy dish.

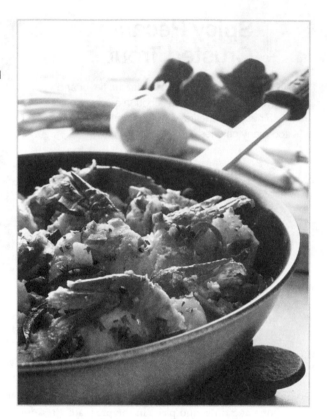

¼   c cornstarch
½   tsp salt
1   lb jumbo shrimp, peeled and
    deveined
1   Tbsp vegetable oil
4   scallions, coarsely chopped
1   sm red or yellow bell pepper, cut
    into slivers
2   Tbsp chopped fresh cilantro or
    parsley
2   cloves garlic, minced
1   serrano chile pepper, seeded and
    chopped (wear plastic gloves when
    handling)
1   Tbsp lime juice
3   Tbsp water
1   tsp sugar
¾   tsp crushed black peppercorns

1. In a shallow bowl, combine the cornstarch and salt. Add the shrimp. Toss to coat.
2. Heat the oil in a large nonstick skillet over medium–high heat. Add the shrimp, and cook for
   1½ minutes per side, or just until opaque. Add the scallions, bell pepper, cilantro, garlic, and
   chile pepper. Cook, stirring often, for 1 minute. Add the lime juice, water, sugar, and peppercorns.
   Cook, stirring constantly, for 1 minute, or until the shrimp are opaque.

Makes 4 servings

Per serving: 164 cal, 18 g pro, 12 g carb, 4 g fat, 1 g sat. fat, 161 mg chol, 1 g fiber, 483 mg sodium
Diet exchanges: 0 milk, ½ vegetable, 0 fruit, ½ bread, 2½ meat, ½ fat

‖ Crab Cakes

Reduced-fat mayonnaise and egg whites keep the fat at bay in these tender cakes. Browning in a nonstick skillet instead of deep-frying reduces the fat even further.

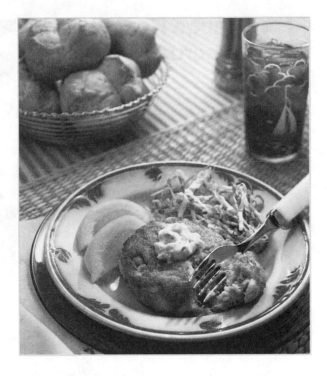

12	**chowder or soda crackers, crushed (about 1 c)**
2	**egg whites**
1	**Tbsp Worcestershire sauce**
2	**tsp crab-boil seasoning**
6	**Tbsp reduced-fat mayonnaise**
1	**lb lump crabmeat**
1	**tsp pickle relish**
1	**tsp minced onion**
4	**lemon wedges**

1. In a large bowl, combine the crackers, egg whites, Worcestershire, crab-boil seasoning, and 2 tablespoons of the mayonnaise. Gently fold in the crabmeat. Form into 4 patties.
2. Heat a large skillet coated with cooking spray over medium heat. Add the crab cakes, and cook for 20 minutes, turning once, or until crispy.
3. In a small bowl, combine the relish, onion, and the remaining 4 tablespoons mayonnaise. Serve the crab cakes with the sauce and lemon wedges.

Makes 4 servings

‖ **Per serving:** 270 cal, 27 g pro, 16 g carb, 10 g fat, 2 g sat. fat, 88 mg chol, 1 g fiber, 1,012 mg sodium
Diet exchanges: 0 milk, 0 vegetable, 0 fruit, 1 bread, 3½ meat, 1½ fat

Orange Roughy Veracruz

If fish is a new taste for your family, serve dishes with a flavorful sauce such as this Veracruz. For a slight twist, use different flavors of diced tomatoes.

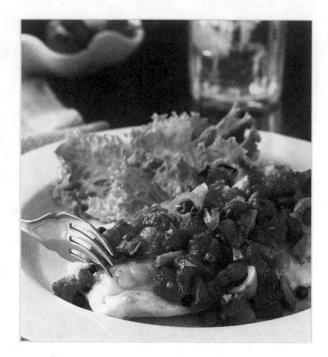

4	orange roughy or red snapper fillets (6 oz each)
1	Tbsp lime juice
1	tsp dried oregano
2	tsp olive oil
1	onion, chopped
1	clove garlic, minced
1	can (15 oz) Mexican-style diced tomatoes
12	pimiento-stuffed olives, coarsely chopped
2	Tbsp chopped parsley

1. Preheat the oven to 350°F. Coat an 8" x 8" baking dish with cooking spray. Place the fillets in the dish. Sprinkle with the lime juice and oregano. Set aside.
2. Heat the oil in a medium skillet over medium heat. Add the onion and garlic, and cook, stirring, for 5 minutes, or until soft. Add the tomatoes (with juice), olives, and parsley. Cook, stirring occasionally, for 5 minutes, or until thickened. Spoon over the fillets. Cover with foil.
3. Bake for 18 to 20 minutes, or until the fish flakes easily.

Makes 4 servings

Per serving: 208 cal, 27 g pro, 14 g carb, 6 g fat, 0 g sat. fat, 34 mg chol, 3 g fiber, 822 mg sodium
Diet exchanges: 0 milk, 2 vegetable, 0 fruit, 0 bread, 3½ meat, 1 fat

Pasta with Beans and Cajun Salmon

Using beans in this dish adds a nice flavor while increasing the fiber content. Canned beans are good to keep on hand to stir into many of your favorite dishes.

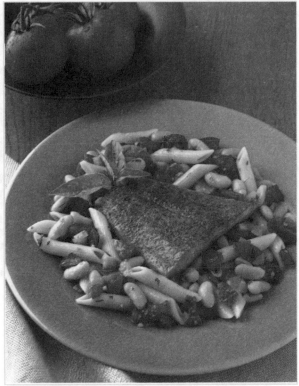

½	**lb penne**
1	**onion, chopped**
2	**cloves garlic, minced**
6	**plum tomatoes, chopped**
⅓	**c chopped fresh basil**
1	**can (15 oz) cannellini beans, rinsed and drained**
1½	**c fat-free chicken broth**
1	**salmon fillet (1 lb), skinned and cut into 6 pieces**
½	**tsp Cajun seasoning**

1. Prepare the pasta per package directions. Drain, and return to the pot.
2. Meanwhile, heat a large nonstick skillet coated with cooking spray over medium heat. Add the onion and garlic, and cook, stirring, for 5 minutes, or until soft. Add the tomatoes and basil, and cook, stirring occasionally, for 4 minutes. Add the beans and broth, and simmer for 4 minutes, or until slightly reduced. Stir into the pasta, and keep warm.
3. Coat both sides of the salmon with cooking spray. Sprinkle with the Cajun seasoning. Wipe the skillet with paper towels, then heat over medium-high heat. Add the salmon, and cook for 4 minutes per side, or until the fish flakes easily.
4. To serve, evenly divide the pasta mixture among six plates. Top each serving with a salmon fillet.

Makes 6 servings

Per serving: 401 cal, 32 g pro, 39 g carb, 13 g fat, 3 g sat. fat, 67 mg chol, 5 g fiber, 334 mg sodium
Diet exchanges: 0 milk, 1 vegetable, 0 fruit, 2 bread, 3½ meat, ½ fat

Chili-Spiced Beef Stew

This beef stew is made healthier by using only 4 oz of meat per serving and increasing the vegetables.

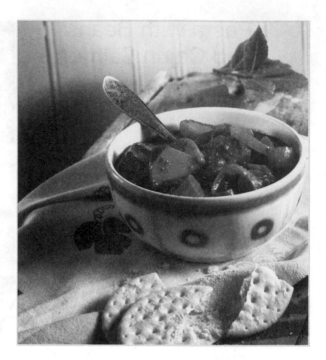

2	Tbsp whole grain pastry flour
4	tsp chili powder
½	tsp salt
2	lb beef stew meat
1	Tbsp olive oil
2	onions, sliced
3	cloves garlic, minced
1	tsp dried oregano
2	c beef broth
2	cans (14 oz each) stewed tomatoes
1	tsp sugar
2	potatoes, cubed
4	carrots, sliced ½" thick

1. In a large resealable plastic bag, combine the flour, 1½ teaspoons of the chili powder, and the salt. Add the beef, seal the bag, and toss to coat well.
2. Heat the oil in a large saucepan over medium–high heat. Add the beef, and cook, stirring occasionally, for 7 minutes, or until browned. Add the onions, garlic, and oregano. Reduce the heat to medium, and cook, stirring often, for 5 minutes.
3. Add the broth, tomatoes, sugar, and the remaining 2½ teaspoons chili powder. Bring to a boil. Reduce the heat to low, cover, and simmer for 2 hours, or until the beef is almost tender, stirring occasionally.
4. Add the potatoes and carrots. Cook, covered, for 30 minutes, or until the vegetables are tender.

Makes 8 servings

Per serving: 269 cal, 28 g pro, 25 g carb, 7 g fat, 2 g sat. fat, 69 mg chol, 4 g fiber, 629 mg sodium
Diet exchanges: 0 milk, 2½ vegetable, 0 fruit, ½ bread, 3½ meat, 1 fat

‖ Beef Stroganoff

The leanest cuts of beef make for healthier dishes. Cuts with the word "round" or "loin" in their name are the best—so choose eye of round, top round, sirloin, or tenderloin.

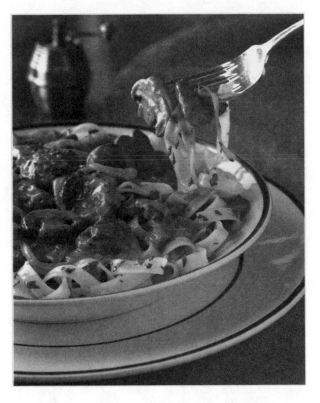

12	oz med no-yolk egg noodles
1	tsp vegetable oil
¾	lb beef tenderloin or top round, trimmed of all visible fat and cut crosswise into thin strips
1	sm onion, quartered and thinly sliced
½	lb mushrooms, stems removed and caps sliced
1½	Tbsp unbleached flour
1	can (14½ oz) fat-free beef broth
1	tsp Worcestershire sauce
¼	c reduced-fat sour cream
2	Tbsp chopped fresh parsley

1. Prepare the noodles per package directions. Drain, and place in a serving bowl.
2. Heat the oil in a large nonstick skillet over medium-high heat. Add the beef, and cook, turning occasionally, for 3 minutes, or until browned. Remove to a plate.
3. Coat the skillet with cooking spray. Reduce the heat to medium. Add the onion, and cook, stirring, for 3 minutes. Add the mushrooms, and cook, stirring, for 3 minutes, or until they begin to release liquid. Sprinkle with the flour, and cook, stirring constantly, for 1 minute.
4. Add the broth and Worcestershire sauce, and cook, stirring, for 3 minutes, or until slightly thickened. Remove from the heat, and stir in the sour cream and parsley. Return the beef to the skillet. Place over low heat, and cook for 3 minutes, or until heated through.
5. Serve the stroganoff over the noodles.

Makes 6 servings

‖ **Per serving:** 351 cal, 18 g pro, 35 g carb, 16 g fat, 6 g sat. fat, 43 mg chol, 3 g fiber, 377 mg sodium
Diet exchanges: 0 milk, ½ vegetable, 0 fruit, 2 bread, 1½ meat, 1 fat

Spaghetti with Meatballs

Your family will love these flavorful meatballs—and you'll love the reduced fat and calories that come from combining ground turkey breast with ground beef.

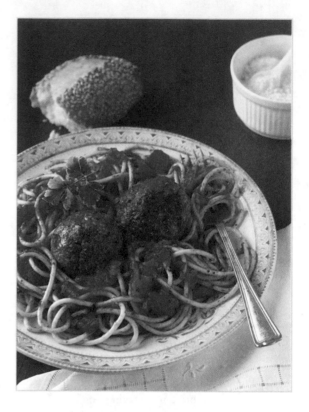

2	onions, chopped
3	cloves garlic, minced
½	lb extra-lean ground round beef
½	lb ground turkey breast
⅔	c fresh bread crumbs
¼	c fat-free milk
1	egg, lightly beaten
2	tsp Italian seasoning
¼	tsp salt
2	tsp olive oil
2	cans (15 oz each) tomato sauce
1	can (15 oz) diced tomatoes
2	Tbsp sugar
2	Tbsp Italian seasoning
¾	lb spaghetti

1. Heat a Dutch oven coated with cooking spray over medium heat. Add the onions and garlic, and cook, stirring occasionally, for 6 minutes, or until soft. Remove ¼ cup of the onion mixture to a large bowl. Place the remaining mixture in a small bowl.

2. Combine the beef, turkey, bread crumbs, milk, egg, Italian seasoning, and salt in the large bowl with the onions. Shape into 12 meatballs.

3. Coat the same Dutch oven with cooking spray. Add the oil, and heat over medium-high heat. Add the meatballs, and cook, turning, for 5 minutes, or until well browned.

4. Add the tomato sauce, diced tomatoes (with juice), sugar, Italian seasoning, and the reserved onion mixture. Bring to a boil over high heat. Reduce the heat to low. Cover and simmer, stirring occasionally, for 20 minutes, or until the meatballs are cooked through.

5. Meanwhile, prepare the pasta per package directions. Place in a serving bowl. Top with the sauce and meatballs.

Makes 6 servings

Per serving: 478 cal, 28 g pro, 68 g carb, 10 g fat, 3 g sat. fat, 6 g fiber, 79 mg chol, 954 mg sodium
Diet exchanges: 0 milk, 3 vegetable, 0 fruit, 3 bread, 2 meat, ½ fat

‖ Confetti Meat Loaf

Brown rice and chopped vegetables combine with ground beef or turkey to add fiber, vitamins, and minerals to this tasty meat loaf.

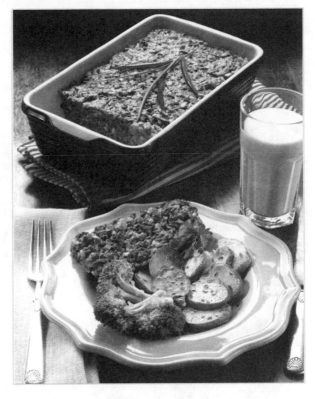

½	c brown rice
1	Tbsp olive oil or vegetable oil
1	sm onion, chopped
2	red and/or green bell peppers, chopped
1	lb extra-lean ground beef and/or ground turkey breast
1	c chunky salsa
1	egg
¾	tsp salt
½	tsp ground black pepper

1. Prepare the rice per package directions. Preheat the oven to 350°F.
2. Heat the oil in a small skillet over medium heat. Add the onion and bell peppers, and cook for 5 minutes, or until tender.
3. In a large bowl, combine the meat, salsa, egg, salt, and black pepper. Add the vegetables and rice. Place the mixture in a roasting pan, and pat into an oblong loaf. Bake for 45 minutes, or until a meat thermometer inserted in the center registers 160°F and the meat is no longer pink.

Makes 6 servings

Per serving: 246 cal, 18 g pro, 18 g carb, 10 g fat, 3 g sat. fat, 63 mg chol, 1 g fiber, 665 mg sodium
Diet exchanges: 0 milk, 1 vegetable, 0 fruit, 1 bread, 2½ meat, ½ fat

Super-Stuffed Potatoes

Using turkey bacon in these stuffed potatoes adds a smoky flavor while keeping fat and calories at healthy levels.

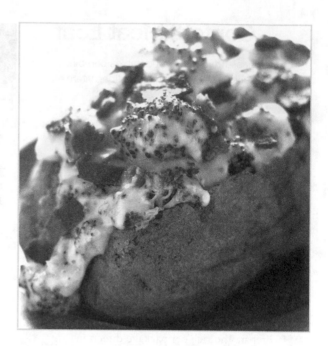

4	russet potatoes
1	Tbsp unbleached flour
⅛	tsp ground nutmeg
1	c + ⅔ c 1% milk
1	c shredded reduced-fat extra-sharp Cheddar cheese
¼	tsp salt
1	pkg (10 oz) frozen chopped broccoli, thawed and drained
3	strips turkey bacon, chopped and cooked until crisp

1. Preheat the oven to 425°F. Pierce the potatoes several times with a fork. Place in the oven, and bake for 1 hour, or until tender.

2. Meanwhile, in a small saucepan, combine the flour and nutmeg. Gradually whisk in 1 cup of the milk until the flour dissolves. Cook, stirring, over medium heat for 5 minutes, or until thickened. Remove from the heat. Stir in the cheese until smooth. Set aside.

3. Holding the potatoes with an oven mitt, cut in half lengthwise. Scoop the flesh out into a bowl, leaving a ¼" shell. Place the shells on a baking sheet coated with cooking spray. Mash the flesh with a potato masher. Stir in the remaining ⅔ cup milk and the salt until smooth. Spoon the potato mixture into the shells. Top with the broccoli, bacon, and cheese sauce. Bake for 10 minutes, or until heated through.

Makes 8 servings

Per serving: 139 cal, 10 g pro, 19 g carb, 4 g fat, 2 g sat. fat, 18 mg chol, 3 g fiber, 277 mg sodium
Diet exchanges: 0 milk, ½ vegetable, 0 fruit, ½ bread, ½ meat, ½ fat

Buttermilk-Herb Mashed Potatoes

These creamy mashed potatoes are a good source of calcium and a perfect accompaniment to almost any meal. Low-fat buttermilk and nonfat sour cream keep the fat content down.

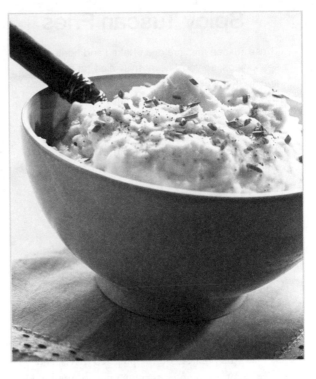

3	lb Yukon gold potatoes, cut into 1" cubes
1½	c buttermilk
¾	c nonfat sour cream
1	Tbsp chopped fresh Italian parsley
1	Tbsp chopped fresh chives
⅛	tsp salt
⅛	tsp ground black pepper

1. Place the potatoes in a large saucepan. Cover with water, and bring to a boil over high heat. Reduce the heat to medium, and cook for 15 minutes, or until the potatoes are tender. Drain, and return to the saucepan. Mash with a potato masher until almost smooth.

2. Add the buttermilk, sour cream, parsley, chives, salt, and pepper. Cook over medium heat for 3 minutes, or until hot.

Makes 6 servings

Per serving: 199 cal, 9 g pro, 46 g carb, 1 g fat, 0 g sat. fat, 2 mg chol, 5 g fiber, 167 mg sodium
Diet exchanges: ½ milk, 0 vegetable, 0 fruit, 2 bread, 0 meat, 0 fat

‖ Spicy Tuscan Fries

These Tuscan fries are oven-baked and coated with seasonings, so you'll never miss high-fat french fries again. After washing, don't peel the potatoes—that way you'll retain the valuable nutrients found in and next to the skin.

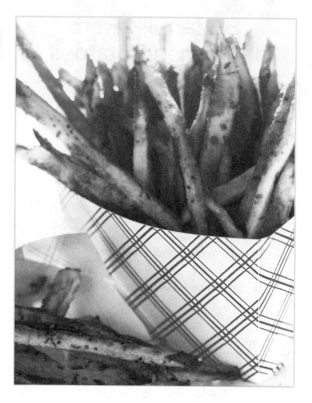

4	russet potatoes, cut into ¼" slices
2	Tbsp grated Parmesan cheese
1	tsp dried basil
½	tsp salt
¼	tsp ground black pepper
¼	tsp ground red pepper

1. Preheat the oven to 425°F. Coat two baking sheets with cooking spray.
2. Place the potatoes in a large bowl, and coat with cooking spray. Sprinkle with the cheese, basil, salt, and peppers. Toss to mix well.
3. Place the potatoes on the prepared sheets, and bake for 25 minutes, turning once, or until tender.

Makes 4 servings

Per serving: 116 cal, 5 g pro, 26 g carb, 1 g fat, 1 g sat. fat, 2 mg chol, 3 g fiber, 349 mg sodium
Diet exchanges: 0 milk, 0 vegetable, 0 fruit, 1½ bread, 0 meat, 0 fat

Stuffed Acorn Squash

Barley is a high-fiber grain that adds a nutty flavor to stuffing. For a faster dinner, opt for the quick-cooking variety.

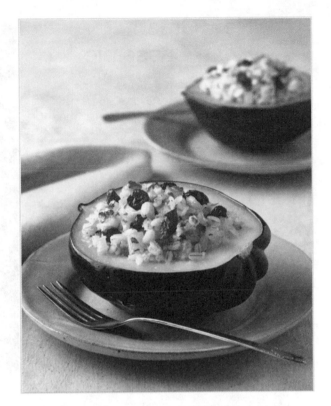

⅔	c pearled barley
3	acorn squash, halved lengthwise, seeds removed
2	tsp vegetable oil
1	sm onion, chopped
1	rib celery, chopped
1	clove garlic, chopped
3	oz mushrooms, sliced
¼	c chopped fresh herb such as thyme, sage, or parsley, or 2 tsp dried
1	c coarse fresh bread crumbs
⅔	c dried cranberries
1	tsp grated lemon peel
¼	tsp salt
¼–½	c vegetable broth or apple juice

1. Prepare the barley per package directions.
2. Preheat the oven to 400°F. Place the squash, cut side up, in a roasting pan. Coat the cut sides lightly with cooking spray. Bake for 30 minutes, or until fork-tender.
3. Meanwhile, heat the oil in a medium nonstick skillet over medium heat. Add the onion, celery, and garlic, and cook for 2 minutes. Add the mushrooms and herb, and cook for 4 minutes, or until the mushrooms are soft. Remove from the heat. Stir in the bread crumbs, cranberries, lemon peel, salt, and barley. Add up to ½ cup broth to moisten and bind the stuffing.
4. Spoon the stuffing into the squash halves. Bake for 10 minutes, or until heated through.

Makes 6 servings

Per serving: 256 cal, 6 g pro, 56 g carb, 2 g fat, 0 g sat. fat, 0 mg chol, 9 g fiber, 200 mg sodium
Diet exchanges: 0 milk, 4 vegetable, ½ fruit, 1½ bread, 0 meat, ½ fat

New Green Bean Casserole

A delicious take on the high-fat classic, this dish is sure to become a family favorite. Homemade oven-baked onion rings are simple to make and taste delicious.

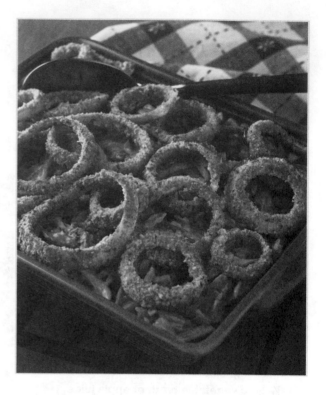

½	c buttermilk
½	c plain dry bread crumbs
1	med onion, cut crosswise into ¼"-thick slices and separated into rings
2	tsp olive oil
½	lb mushrooms, sliced
1	sm onion, chopped
¼	c unbleached flour
½	tsp dried thyme
¼	tsp salt
3	c 1% milk
1	bag (16 oz) frozen french-cut green beans, thawed and drained

1. Preheat the oven to 500°F. Coat a 3-quart baking dish and a baking sheet with cooking spray.
2. Place the buttermilk in a shallow bowl. Place the bread crumbs in another shallow bowl. Dip the onion rings into the buttermilk, dredge in the bread crumbs, and place on a baking sheet. Coat with cooking spray. Bake for 20 minutes, or until tender and golden brown.
3. Meanwhile, heat the oil in a medium saucepan over medium heat. Add the mushrooms and onion, and cook, stirring, for 5 minutes, or until the mushrooms give off liquid. Sprinkle with the flour, thyme, and salt. Cook, stirring, for 1 minute. Add the milk, and cook, stirring constantly, for 3 minutes, or until thickened. Stir in the green beans.
4. Reduce the oven to 400°F. Place the bean mixture in the prepared baking dish. Place the onion rings over the top. Bake for 25 minutes, or until hot and bubbly.

Makes 8 servings

Per serving: 136 cal, 8 g pro, 22 g carb, 3 g fat, 1 g sat. fat, 6 mg chol, 3 g fiber, 199 mg sodium
Diet exchanges: ½ milk, 1½ vegetable, 0 fruit, ½ bread, 0 meat, ½ fat

Broccoli-Cheese Spoon Bread

This rich spoon bread is a source of calcium but not fat, thanks to fat-free evaporated milk and reduced-fat cheese. You can use less cheese by choosing an extra-sharp variety, which packs the most flavor.

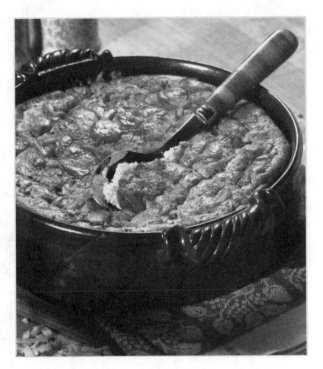

1	can (7 oz) fat-free evaporated milk
½	c yellow cornmeal
½	tsp sugar
¼	tsp ground black pepper
½	c shredded reduced-fat extra-sharp Cheddar cheese
2	lg eggs
2	lg egg whites
1	box (10 oz) frozen chopped broccoli, thawed and drained
¼	c chopped roasted red peppers
¼	tsp salt

1. Preheat the oven to 375°F. Coat a 2-quart baking dish with cooking spray.
2. Place the evaporated milk in a medium saucepan over medium heat. Gradually add the cornmeal, and cook, stirring constantly, for 3 minutes, or until thickened. Remove from the heat, and stir in the sugar, black pepper, and 6 tablespoons of the cheese until the cheese melts.
3. Beat the whole eggs in a small bowl. Add ¼ cup of the hot milk mixture to the eggs, stirring constantly. Stir the egg mixture into the remaining milk mixture.
4. In a medium bowl, beat the egg whites until stiff. Fold into the milk mixture. Fold in the broccoli, roasted peppers, and salt. Pour into the prepared baking dish. Bake for 50 minutes, or until a knife inserted in the center comes out clean. Sprinkle with the remaining 2 tablespoons cheese.

Makes 4 servings

Per serving: 207 cal, 16 g pro, 24 g carb, 6 g fat, 2 g sat. fat, 120 mg chol, 3 g fiber, 392 mg sodium
Diet exchanges: ½ milk, ½ vegetable, 0 fruit, 1 bread, 1 meat, ½ fat

Molasses Baked Beans

Beans are a great source of fiber and should be included in your diet several times a week. But convenient canned beans are packed with sodium, so be sure to always rinse them to remove one-third of the added salt.

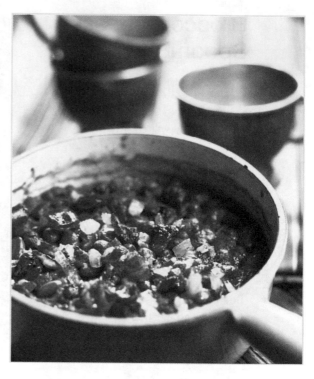

3	cans (15 oz each) pinto beans
1	strip bacon, chopped
1	sm onion, chopped
½	c barbecue sauce
½	c molasses
1	Tbsp brown mustard
2	tsp Worcestershire sauce

1. Preheat the oven to 350°F. Coat a 2-quart baking dish with cooking spray.
2. Drain the beans, reserving ½ cup of the liquid. Rinse and drain the beans.
3. In a large skillet, cook the bacon, stirring, for 3 minutes, or until crisp. Remove with a slotted spoon to a paper towel. Add the onion, and cook, stirring, for 5 minutes, or until soft.
4. Remove from the heat, and stir in the beans, reserved liquid, barbecue sauce, molasses, mustard, and Worcestershire.
5. Place in the prepared dish, and bake for 30 minutes, or until heated through.

Makes 6 servings

Per serving: 313 cal, 12 g pro, 57 g carb, 4 g fat, 1 g sat. fat, 3 mg chol, 12 g fiber, 788 mg sodium
Diet exchanges: 0 milk, ½ vegetable, 0 fruit, 3½ bread, 0 meat, ½ fat

‖ Healthy Coleslaw

Most people don't realize that cabbage is a very nutritious food. Making coleslaw is probably the easiest way to get its healing properties.

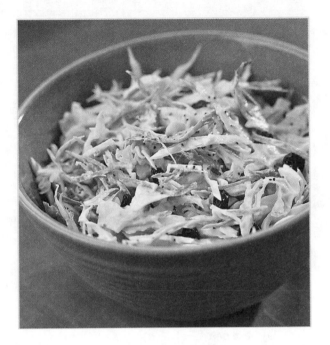

Dressing

1	c fat-free plain yogurt
¼	c apple cider vinegar
1	Tbsp honey

Slaw

1	lb (1 sm head) green cabbage, shredded
½	c shredded carrots
1	Tbsp poppy seeds
¼	c raisins or currants

In a large bowl, combine the dressing ingredients. Add the cabbage, carrots, poppy seeds, and raisins. Mix well until the dressing completely coats the cabbage.

Makes 8 servings

From The Diabetes Food & Nutrition Bible: A Complete Guide to Planning, Shopping, Cooking, and Eating *by Hope Warshaw, MMSc, RD, CDE, and Robyn Webb, MS (American Diabetes Association, 2001; $18.95/trade paperback)*

Per serving: 58 cal, 3 g pro, 12 g carb, 1 g fat, 0 g sat. fat, 1 mg chol, 2 g fiber, 36 mg sodium
Diet exchanges: 0 milk, 0 vegetable, 0 fruit, 1 bread, 0 meat, 0 fat

CHAPTER 21

Dessert

Craving an after-dinner indulgence? Here are 16 mouthwatering treats that won't derail your blood sugar

‖ Pecan Coffee Cake

Fat-free sour cream adds richness without adding fat and calories. The whole grain pastry flour provides a bit of fiber, making this cake a guilt-free treat.

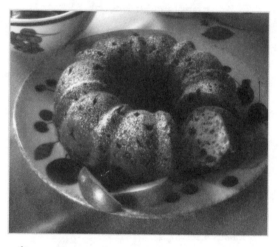

1½	**c whole grain pastry flour**
2	**tsp baking powder**
½	**tsp baking soda**
½	**tsp salt**
¼	**tsp ground cinnamon**
½	**c packed brown sugar**
2	**Tbsp butter or margarine, softened**
¾	**c liquid egg substitute**
½	**c fat-free sour cream**
½	**c raisins**

½	**c chopped pecans**
½	**Tbsp confectioners' sugar**

1. Preheat the oven to 350°F. Coat an 8" Bundt pan with cooking spray.
2. In a medium bowl, combine the flour, baking powder, baking soda, salt, and cinnamon.
3. In a large bowl, with an electric mixer on low speed, beat the brown sugar and butter until smooth. Beat in the egg substitute and sour cream.
4. Gradually beat in the flour mixture until the batter is smooth. Stir in the raisins and pecans.
5. Place the batter in the prepared pan, and bake for 35 minutes, or until a wooden pick inserted in the center comes out clean. Cool for 10 minutes on a rack. Remove from the pan, and cool completely. Sprinkle with the confectioners' sugar just before serving.

Makes 9 servings

Per serving: 218 cal, 6 g pro, 31 g carb, 9 g fat, 2 g sat. fat, 8 mg chol, 3 g fiber, 366 mg sodium
Diet exchanges: 0 milk, 0 vegetable, 0 fruit, 2 bread, ½ meat, 1½ fat

‖ Chocolate Soufflé Cake

Fat-free sour cream takes the place of some of the butter in this recipe, reducing the fat and calories while adding a rich flavor.

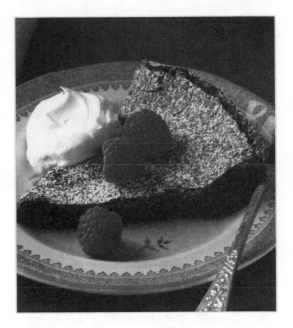

½	tsp + 1 Tbsp unbleached flour
2	oz semisweet chocolate, melted and cooled slightly
2	Tbsp butter or margarine, softened
5	Tbsp fat-free sour cream
1	egg yolk
¼	tsp vanilla extract
1	c granulated sugar
3	Tbsp cocoa powder
4	egg whites, at room temperature
⅛	tsp cream of tartar
2	Tbsp confectioners' sugar

1. Preheat the oven to 350°F. Coat an 8" springform pan with cooking spray. Dust with ½ teaspoon of the flour.
2. In a medium bowl, combine the melted chocolate, butter, sour cream, egg yolk, vanilla extract, and ¾ cup of the granulated sugar, stirring until well blended. Fold in the cocoa and the remaining 1 tablespoon flour.
3. In a large bowl, combine the egg whites and cream of tartar. With an electric mixer on medium speed, beat until soft peaks form. Increase the speed to high. Beat, gradually adding the remaining ¼ cup granulated sugar, until stiff peaks form. Fold about one-third of the egg white mixture into the chocolate mixture. Gently fold in the remaining egg white mixture. Spoon into the prepared pan.
4. Bake for 30 minutes, or until a wooden pick inserted in the center comes out with just a few moist crumbs. Cool on a rack. The cake will fall as it cools, leaving a raised edge. Gently press down on the edge as it cools.
5. To serve, remove the pan's side, and place the cake on a serving plate. Sift the confectioners' sugar over the cake.

Makes 10 servings

Per serving: 155 cal, 3 g pro, 27 g carb, 5 g fat, 3 g sat. fat, 27 mg chol, 1 g fiber, 56 mg sodium
Diet exchanges: 0 milk, 0 vegetable, 0 fruit, 1½ bread, 0 meat, 1 fat

Chocolate-Cherry Bread Pudding

Whole wheat bread boosts the fiber content of this homestyle dessert. Prune puree replaces the butter to cut down on fat and calories while adding even more fiber.

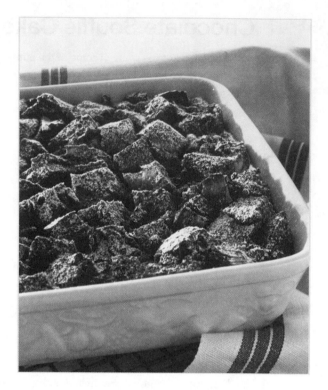

8	oz thick-sliced whole wheat bread, cut into cubes (about 5½ c)
½	c dried sour cherries
½	c boiling water
⅔	c packed brown sugar
⅓	c cocoa powder
3½	c 1% milk
4	egg whites, lightly beaten
¾	c prune puree
2	tsp vanilla extract
1	oz semisweet chocolate, finely chopped
1	Tbsp confectioners' sugar

1. Preheat the oven to 350°F. Coat a medium baking dish with cooking spray. Place the bread cubes in the dish.
2. Place the cherries in a small bowl, and cover with the boiling water. Let stand for 5 minutes, or until the cherries are plump. Drain any remaining water.
3. In a large bowl, whisk together the brown sugar, cocoa, milk, egg whites, prune puree, and vanilla extract. Stir in the chocolate and cherries. Pour over the bread cubes. Press down lightly to moisten all of the bread. Let stand for 15 minutes for the bread to absorb the liquid.
4. Bake for 40 minutes, or until slightly puffed and set. Remove from the oven, and cool slightly. Sift the confectioners' sugar over the pudding.

Makes 10 servings

Per serving: 215 cal, 8 g pro, 41 g carb, 3 g fat, 2 g sat. fat, 3 mg chol, 3 g fiber, 193 mg sodium
Diet exchanges: ½ milk, 0 vegetable, ½ fruit, 2 bread, 0 meat, 0 fat

Lemon-Scented Bread Pudding

Typically made with half-and-half, this healthier version of bread pudding uses 1% milk to keep a creamy flavor without a lot of fat and calories.

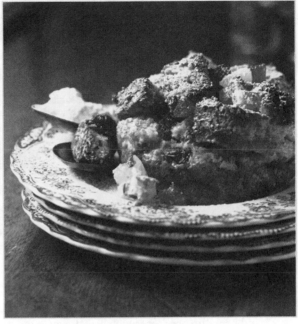

8	oz French or Italian bread, cut into cubes (about 5½ c)
1½	c 1% milk
½	c sugar
1	Tbsp lemon peel
3	eggs
1	tsp vanilla extract
	Fresh raspberries and/or blueberries

1. Coat a 9" x 5" loaf pan with cooking spray. Place the bread cubes in the prepared pan.
2. In a small saucepan over low heat, combine the milk, sugar, and lemon peel. Cook, stirring occasionally, until the sugar is dissolved. Remove from the heat, and let stand for 15 minutes.
3. In a large bowl, whisk together the eggs and vanilla extract. Slowly whisk in the milk mixture. Pour over the bread, and press down lightly to make sure that all of the bread is moistened. Cover, and refrigerate for 2 hours.
4. Preheat the oven to 350°F. Uncover the bread pudding, and press down lightly on the bread to coat with filling. Bake for 35 minutes, or until slightly puffed and set. If the top browns too quickly, cover with foil during the last 15 minutes of baking time. Cool on a rack for at least 20 minutes. Serve warm, or cover and refrigerate for at least 3 hours. Serve with the berries.

Makes 8 servings

Per serving: 184 cal, 7 g pro, 32 g carb, 3 g fat, 1 g sat. fat, 81 mg chol, 2 g fiber, 219 mg sodium
Diet exchanges: 0 milk, 0 vegetable, 0 fruit, 2 bread, ½ meat, 0 fat

Hearty Rice Pudding

Brown rice and fat-free milk turn this rice pudding into a healthy treat the whole family will love. In fact, brown rice substitutes perfectly for white rice in any recipe—and it adds health-boosting fiber and vitamins.

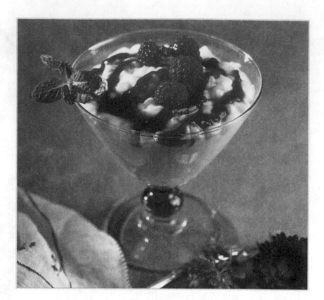

3	c fat-free milk
½	c uncooked brown rice
¼	c + 1 tsp brown sugar
⅛	tsp salt
1	tsp vanilla extract
2	eggs, lightly beaten
½	pint fresh raspberries

1. In a medium saucepan, combine the milk, rice, ¼ cup of the sugar, salt, and vanilla extract, and bring to a boil over high heat. Reduce the heat to low, cover, and simmer for 1½ hours. Remove from the heat, and let cool for 5 minutes.
2. Stir ½ cup of the rice mixture into the eggs. Gradually stir the egg mixture into the saucepan.
3. Place over medium-low heat, and cook, stirring constantly, for 5 minutes, or until thickened. Cool for 10 minutes to serve warm. Or place in a bowl, cover with plastic wrap, and refrigerate for at least 3 hours.
4. Reserve half of the raspberries for garnish. In a blender, puree the remaining raspberries. Strain to remove the seeds, and stir in the remaining 1 teaspoon sugar.
5. To serve, spoon the pudding into dessert dishes, drizzle with the raspberry sauce, and top with the remaining raspberries.

Makes 8 servings

Per serving: 122 cal, 6 g pro, 20 g carb, 2 g fat, 1 g sat. fat, 55 mg chol, 1 g fiber, 112 mg sodium
Diet exchanges: ½ milk, 0 vegetable, 0 fruit, 1 bread, 0 meat, 0 fat

Pear-Oatmeal Crumble

Here's a great way to add healthy oatmeal to your diet. Leave the skin on the pears to get the most fiber and nutrients.

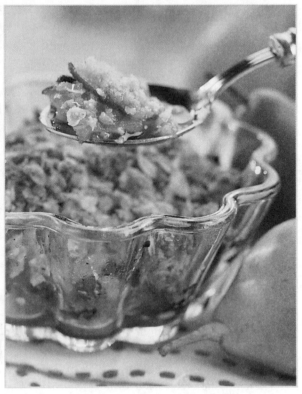

½	**c rolled oats**
¼	**c whole grain pastry flour**
2	**Tbsp packed brown sugar**
1	**tsp ground cinnamon**
2	**Tbsp cold butter or margarine, cut into small pieces**
3	**lg Bosc pears, cored and thinly sliced**
¼	**c frozen apple juice concentrate, thawed**
3	**Tbsp dried currants**
1	**Tbsp honey**
1	**tsp lemon juice**

1. Preheat the oven to 400°F. Coat a 9" x 9" baking dish with cooking spray.
2. In a medium bowl, combine the oats, flour, sugar, and ½ teaspoon of the cinnamon. Using your fingers or a pastry blender, lightly mix in the butter until coarse crumbs form.
3. In another medium bowl, combine the pears, apple juice concentrate, currants, honey, lemon juice, and the remaining ½ teaspoon cinnamon. Place in the prepared dish, and top with the crumb mixture.
4. Bake for 20 minutes, or until the pears are tender and the filling is bubbly.

Makes 6 servings

Per serving: 202 cal, 3 g pro, 40 g carb, 5 g fat, 2 g sat. fat, 10 mg chol, 4 g fiber, 45 mg sodium
Diet exchanges: 0 milk, 0 vegetable, 1½ fruit, 1 bread, 0 meat, 1 fat

‖ Pumpkin Pie

It's often the crust that adds too much fat and calories to a pie. This lower-fat version of an American classic uses reduced-fat cream cheese in place of some of the butter for a tender, flavorful crust.

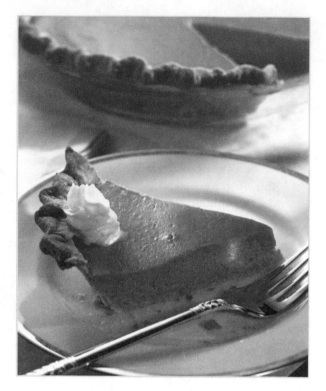

1½	c whole grain pastry flour
½	teaspoon salt
¼	c cold butter or margarine, cut into small pieces
2	Tbsp reduced-fat cream cheese
4	Tbsp ice water
2	eggs
2	c solid-pack canned pumpkin
1	can (12 oz) fat-free evaporated milk
¾	c packed brown sugar
1	tsp vanilla extract
1	tsp ground cinnamon
½	tsp ground ginger
½	tsp ground nutmeg

1. Preheat the oven to 400°F.
2. In a food processor, combine the flour and ¼ teaspoon of the salt. Process to blend. Add the butter and cream cheese, and pulse until the mixture resembles cornmeal. Drizzle 3 tablespoons of the water over the mixture. Pulse until crumbly and the dough forms a ball that will hold together when pressed. Add 1 more tablespoon of water if necessary.
3. Place the dough on a piece of plastic wrap, and press into a disk. Wrap, and chill for 30 minutes. Roll the dough out to an 11" circle. Place in a 9" pie plate. Press the dough into the bottom and sides of the plate. Fold the edges under, and crimp the crust.
4. Lightly beat the eggs in a large bowl. Stir in the pumpkin, evaporated milk, sugar, vanilla extract, cinnamon, ginger, nutmeg, and the remaining ¼ teaspoon salt until well blended. Place in the prepared crust.
5. Bake for 10 minutes. Reduce the oven temperature to 350°F, and bake for 40 minutes, or until a knife inserted in the center comes out clean. Cool on a rack for at least 2 hours. Chill in the refrigerator until ready to serve.

Makes 10 servings

‖ **Per serving:** 240 cal, 7 g pro, 40 g carb, 6 g fat, 4 g sat. fat, 60 mg chol, 5 g fiber, 242 mg sodium
‖ **Diet exchanges:** ½ milk, 0 vegetable, 0 fruit, 2½ bread, ½ meat, 1 fat

Creamy Chocolate Mousse Pie

This guilt-free chocolate dessert comes together in minutes thanks to instant pudding mix made with fat-free milk and light whipped topping. Vanilla extract and espresso powder bring out the rich chocolate flavor.

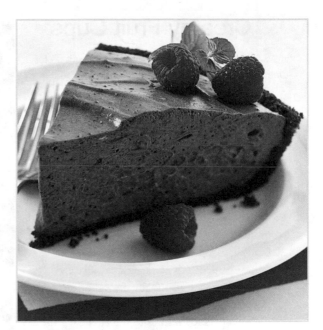

18	chocolate graham crackers
2	Tbsp butter or margarine, melted
2½	c fat-free milk
2	pkg (4 servings each) sugar-free instant chocolate pudding/pie filling
1	tsp vanilla extract
½	tsp instant espresso powder
1	c light whipped topping

1. Preheat the oven to 375°F.
2. Crush the graham crackers into crumbs. In a 9" pie plate, combine the crumbs and butter. Press firmly into the bottom and up the sides of the plate. Bake for 6 minutes. Cool completely on a rack.
3. In a large bowl, whisk together the milk, pudding mix, vanilla extract, and espresso powder for 2 minutes, or until smooth and creamy. Fold in the whipped topping.
4. Spoon into the prepared crust. Cover, and refrigerate for at least 3 hours.

Makes 10 servings

Per serving: 146 cal, 4 g pro, 17 g carb, 7 g fat, 4 g sat. fat, 8 mg chol, 1 g fiber, 173 mg sodium
Diet exchanges: 0 milk, 0 vegetable, 0 fruit, 1 bread, 0 meat, 1 fat

‖ Creamy Fruit Cups

Low-fat wonton wrappers are a great substitute for pastry shells, which are laden with saturated fat.

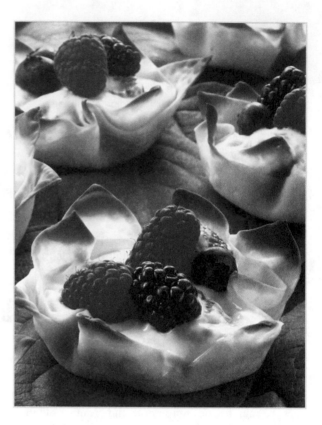

24	wonton wrappers
1¼	c fresh blueberries, blackberries, or raspberries
1	c (8 oz) low-fat vanilla yogurt
⅓	c strawberry all-fruit spread

1. Preheat the oven to 350°F. Coat a 12-cup muffin pan with cooking spray.
2. Line each cup with a wonton wrapper. Coat each wrapper with cooking spray. Place a second wrapper diagonally on top of each of the first ones, making sure that the points of the wrappers form sides to the cup. Coat the second wrappers with cooking spray. Bake for 10 minutes, or until golden brown. Cool on a rack. Remove from the pan.
3. In a medium bowl, combine 1 cup of the berries, the yogurt, and all-fruit spread. Gently toss to blend.
4. Evenly divide the yogurt mixture among the cups. Top with the remaining ¼ cup berries.

Makes 12 servings

Per serving: 84 cal, 3 g pro, 17 g carb, 1 g fat, 0 g sat. fat, 2 mg chol, 0 g fiber, 107 mg sodium
Diet exchanges: 0 milk, 0 vegetable, 0 fruit, 1 bread, 0 meat, 0 fat

‖ Just Peachy Crisp

Here's a delicious low-fat way to enjoy fresh
peaches and blueberries.

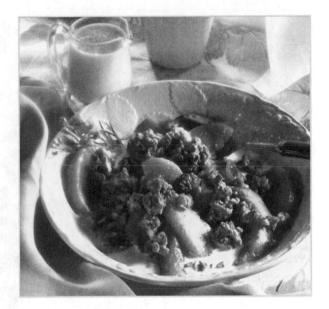

4	med peaches, unpeeled and sliced thin
½	c fresh blueberries
2	tsp lemon juice
1	c water
⅓	c granulated sugar
3	tsp ground cinnamon
1½	Tbsp cornstarch or arrowroot
2	Tbsp flour
¼	c rolled oats
¼	c brown sugar
3	Tbsp canola oil

1. Preheat the oven to 350°F. Coat a baking dish with a little oil.
2. In a saucepan over medium heat, combine the peaches, blueberries, lemon juice, water, granulated sugar, 1 teaspoon of the cinnamon, and cornstarch.
3. Cook over medium heat until the mixture thickens, about 5 to 8 minutes. Pour the hot fruit into the prepared dish.
4. In a small bowl, mix the flour, oats, brown sugar, and the remaining 2 teaspoons cinnamon for the crumb topping. Add the oil, and mix well with a fork. Sprinkle the topping over the peaches. Bake for 10 to 15 minutes, or until the peaches are bubbly and the crisp topping is lightly browned.

Makes 4 servings

From The Diabetes Food & Nutrition Bible: A Complete Guide to Planning, Shopping, Cooking, and Eating *by Hope Warshaw, MMSc, RD, CDE, and Robyn Webb, MS (American Diabetes Association, 2001; $18.95/trade paperback)*

Per serving: 327 cal, 3 g pro, 57 g carb, 11 g fat, 0 g sat. fat, 0 mg chol, 4 g fiber, 7 mg sodium
Diet exchanges: 0 milk, 0 vegetable, 0 fruit, 3½ bread, 0 meat, 2 fat

Oven-Puffed Pancake

Also known as a Dutch Baby, this tender pancake is filled with healthful fruit. Feel free to substitute pears, peaches, or plums for the apples.

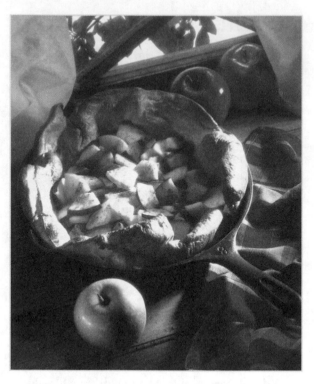

3	apples, coarsely chopped
2	Tbsp packed brown sugar
2	Tbsp lemon juice
¾	c liquid egg substitute
½	c fat-free milk
2	Tbsp canola oil
2	tsp vanilla extract
1	tsp ground nutmeg
½	c unbleached flour

1. Preheat the oven to 450°F. Coat a large ovenproof skillet with cooking spray.
2. In a small bowl, toss the apples with the sugar and lemon juice.
3. In a medium bowl, whisk together the egg substitute, milk, oil, vanilla extract, and nutmeg. Slowly whisk in the flour to form a smooth batter. Pour into the skillet.
4. Cook over medium heat for 2 minutes to set the batter. Bake for 15 minutes. Reduce the oven temperature to 350°F, and bake for 5 minutes, or until puffed and golden brown.
5. Place the apples on top of the pancake, and serve immediately.

Makes 4 servings

Per serving: 279 cal, 10 g pro, 40 g carb, 9 g fat, 1 g sat. fat, 2 mg chol, 4 g fiber, 118 mg sodium
Diet exchanges: 0 milk, 0 vegetable, 1 fruit, 1½ bread, 1 meat, 1½ fat

Roasted Fruit Wraps with Dipping Sauce

This healthy dessert is similar to apple strudel. Healthy whole wheat tortillas substitute for the high-fat, low-fiber phyllo that's layered with butter in traditional strudel.

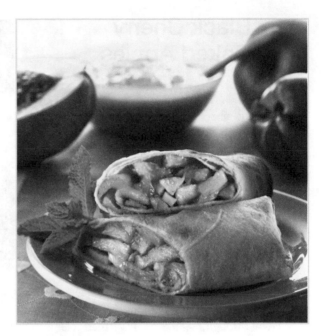

1	c low-fat lemon yogurt
2	tsp finely chopped crystallized ginger
4	Tbsp orange juice
2	Golden Delicious apples, peeled and sliced
3	sm peaches and/or plums, peeled and sliced
4	tsp sugar
⅛	tsp cardamom
4	whole wheat tortillas (8" each)

1. In a small bowl, combine the yogurt, ginger, and 2 tablespoons of the orange juice. Cover, and refrigerate.
2. Preheat the oven to 425°F. Coat a large baking sheet with cooking spray.
3. In a large bowl, combine the apples, peaches, sugar, cardamom, and the remaining 2 tablespoons orange juice. Place on the baking sheet in a single layer. Bake for 10 minutes, or until the fruit is tender.
4. Place one-quarter of the warm fruit down the center of each tortilla. Roll up and place, seam side down, on the baking sheet. Bake for 8 minutes, or until crisp and golden. Cut each wrap in half diagonally. Serve with the yogurt sauce.

Make 4 servings

Per serving: 246 cal, 9 g pro, 48 g carb, 4 g fat, 2 g sat. fat, 3 mg chol, 6 g fiber, 74 mg sodium
Diet exchanges: 0 milk, 0 vegetable, 1 fruit, 2 bread, 0 meat, ½ fat

Black Cherry Baked Apples

Eat your apples with the skin on whenever possible. Besides being a great source of fiber, the skin contains large amounts of quercetin, an antioxidant that helps lower the risk of heart disease and cancer.

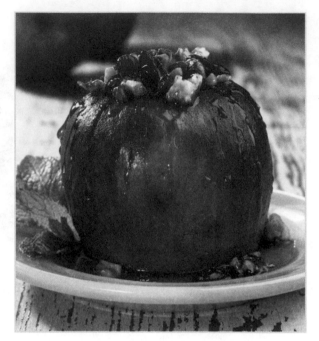

4	**baking apples**
½	**tsp ground cinnamon**
¼	**c dried cherries or raisins**
¼	**c chopped walnuts**
1	**c diet black cherry soda**

1. Preheat the oven to 375°F. Using an apple corer or small knife, remove the apple cores from the stem ends without cutting all the way through the bottom. Place the apples in a 9" x 9" baking dish.

2. Sprinkle the cinnamon inside the apples. Spoon the cherries and walnuts into the apples. Drizzle a little soda into each one. Pour the remaining soda into the baking dish. Bake for 20 minutes, or until tender.

Makes 4 servings

Per serving: 160 cal, 2 g pro, 30 g carb, 5 g fat, 0 g sat. fat, 0 mg chol, 6 g fiber, 9 mg sodium
Diet exchanges: 0 milk, 0 vegetable, 2 fruit, 0 bread, 0 meat, 1 fat

Country-Style Blueberry Muffins

Antioxidant-rich blueberries are extremely flavorful when baked into these fiber-rich muffins.

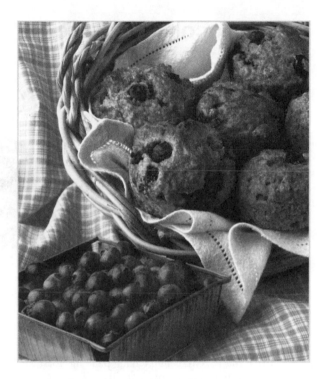

2	**Tbsp + 1½ c whole grain pastry flour**
2	**Tbsp packed brown sugar**
½	**tsp ground cinnamon**
1	**Tbsp cold butter or margarine, cut into small pieces**
½	**c granulated sugar**
2	**tsp baking powder**
½	**tsp salt**
½	**c fat-free milk**
3	**Tbsp fat-free vanilla yogurt**
1	**egg**
1	**Tbsp canola oil**
½	**tsp lemon peel**
1½	**c blueberries**

1. Preheat the oven to 400°F. Coat a 12-cup muffin pan with cooking spray.
2. In a small bowl, combine 2 tablespoons of the flour, the brown sugar, and cinnamon. Using your fingers or a pastry blender, lightly mix in the butter until coarse crumbs form.
3. In a large bowl, combine the granulated sugar, baking powder, salt, and the remaining 1½ cups flour.
4. In a medium bowl, combine the milk, yogurt, egg, oil, and lemon peel. Add to the flour mixture, and stir until just combined. Gently stir in the blueberries.
5. Evenly divide the batter among the muffin cups. Evenly sprinkle the crumb topping over the muffins.
6. Bake for 15 minutes, or until a wooden pick inserted in the center of a muffin comes out clean. Cool on a rack for 5 minutes before removing from the pan.

Makes 12 servings

Per serving: 144 cal, 3 g pro, 27 g carb, 3 g fat, 1 g sat. fat, 21 mg chol, 3 g fiber, 189 mg sodium
Diet exchanges: 0 milk, 0 vegetable, 0 fruit, 1½ bread, 0 meat, ½ fat

Chocolate-Orange Hazelnut Biscotti

When nothing but a cookie will do, these crisp treats are a wise choice. These biscotti are a good source of healthy nuts and are also low in fat and calories.

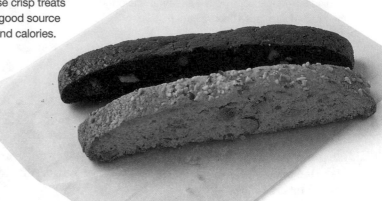

¼	c shelled hazelnuts
2½	c all-purpose flour
¼	c cocoa powder
¾	tsp baking soda
¼	tsp salt
1	c sugar
2	lg eggs
1	lg egg white
1½	tsp grated orange peel
1	tsp vanilla extract

1. Preheat the oven to 350°F. Coat a baking sheet with cooking spray.
2. Place the hazelnuts in a baking pan, and toast for 10 minutes, or until the skins loosen and the nuts are lightly browned. Place the hazelnuts in a kitchen towel, and rub to remove the skins. Finely chop the nuts, and set aside. Reduce the oven temperature to 325°F.
3. In a medium bowl, combine the flour, cocoa, baking soda, and salt.
4. In a large bowl, with an electric mixer at medium speed, beat the sugar, eggs, egg white, orange peel, and vanilla extract until well blended. With the mixer at low speed, gradually add the flour mixture and hazelnuts, and beat until combined.
5. Place the dough on a lightly floured surface. Shape it into two 12" logs.
6. Place the logs on the prepared baking sheet, and bake for 20 minutes, or until the bottoms are lightly browned and the tops are set. Place on a rack to cool slightly, then cut each log diagonally into ½" slices. Return the slices to the baking sheet, and bake for 10 minutes, turning once, or until lightly toasted. Cool completely on a rack.

Makes 40 biscotti

Per biscotti: 58 cal, 2 g pro, 11 g carb, 1 g fat, 0 g sat. fat, 11 mg chol, 1 g fiber, 43 mg sodium
Diet exchanges: 0 milk, 0 vegetable, 0 fruit, ½ bread, 0 meat, 0 fat

Chocolate-Pecan Meringues

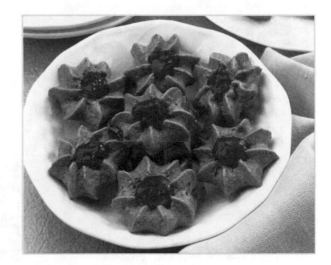

Nuts are an important part of a healthy diet. Here, ground pecans help replace the flour typically used in meringues. For another interesting twist, substitute ground almonds for the pecans.

3	**egg whites**
⅛	**tsp cream of tartar**
⅓	**c sugar**
2	**Tbsp cocoa powder**
¼	**c finely ground pecans**
¼	**c strawberry or raspberry preserves**

1. Preheat the oven to 250°F. Line a baking sheet with parchment or foil.
2. In a large bowl, beat the egg whites until frothy. Add the cream of tartar, and beat until stiff peaks form. Gradually beat the sugar and cocoa into the egg whites. Fold in the pecans.
3. Drop the mixture by spoonfuls on the prepared baking sheet. Using the back of a spoon, depress the centers, and build up the sides of each meringue to form a shallow cup.
4. Bake for 1 hour. Do not open the oven door. Turn off the oven, and let the meringues cool in the oven. Store in an airtight container. When ready to serve, fill each cookie with a heaping ¼ teaspoon of the preserves.

Makes 16 cookies

Per cookie: 45 cal, 1 g pro, 8 g carb, 1 g fat, 0 g sat. fat, 0 mg chol, 0 g fiber, 12 mg sodium
Diet exchanges: 0 milk, 0 vegetable, 0 fruit, ½ bread, 0 meat, 0 fat

CHAPTER 22

Snacks

These nine snacks and sweets aren't just tasty—they're good for you too

‖ Hot Black Bean Dip

Served with baked corn chips, this dip is a healthy alternative to high-fat nachos.

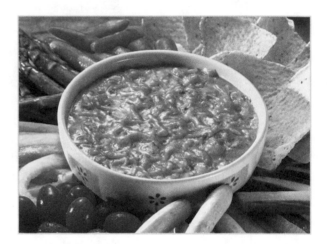

1	can (11 oz) fat-free refried beans
1	c reduced-fat sour cream
1	c salsa
½	tsp salt
1	tsp ground black pepper
½	c shredded reduced-fat Cheddar cheese

1. Preheat the oven to 325°F.
2. In a large bowl, combine the beans, sour cream, salsa, salt, and pepper. Spoon into a shallow 3-cup baking dish. Top with the cheese. Bake for 10 minutes, or until heated through.

Makes 12 servings

‖ **Per serving:** 64 cal, 3 g pro, 8 g carb, 2 g fat, 1 g sat. fat, 7 mg chol, 2 g fiber, 388 mg sodium
Diet exchanges: 0 milk, ½ vegetable, 0 fruit, ½ bread, 0 meat, ½ fat

Vegetable Quesadillas

Flavored cooking sprays add zest to dishes such as these quesadillas while dramatically cutting the fat and calories. Look for a variety of flavors in your supermarket.

1   **sm onion, chopped**
1   **sm zucchini, thinly sliced**
1   **sm yellow squash, thinly sliced**
1   **clove garlic, minced**
1   **can (11 oz) fat-free refried beans**
½   **c shredded reduced-fat Cheddar cheese**
8   **whole wheat tortillas (8" diameter)**
1   **c salsa**

1. Heat a large skillet coated with olive oil spray over medium-high heat. Cook the onion, zucchini, squash, and garlic, stirring, for 7 minutes, or until the vegetables are tender.
2. Evenly divide the vegetables, beans, and cheese over 4 tortillas. Top with the remaining 4 tortillas.
3. Coat the same skillet with cooking spray, and place 1 quesadilla in the skillet. Coat with the spray. Cover, and cook over low heat for 5 minutes, turning once, or until heated through. Repeat with the remaining quesadillas. Cut into wedges. Serve with the salsa.

Makes 4 servings

Per serving: 270 cal, 14 g pro, 59 g carb, 2 g fat, 1 g sat. fat, 5 mg chol, 9 g fiber, 920 mg sodium
Diet exchanges: 0 milk, 1½ vegetable, 0 fruit, 2½ bread, ½ meat, 0 fat

‖ Baked Potato Skins

High-fiber potatoes are an asset to the diabetic diet. Don't peel off the skin—it contains fiber, and most of the potato's nutrients are in the flesh next to the skin.

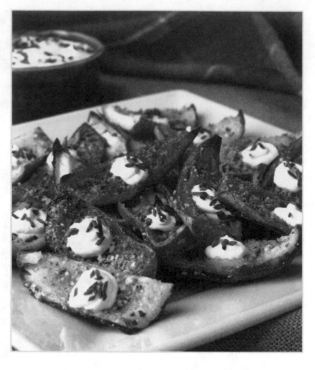

1	lg russet potato
2	lg sweet potatoes
½	c grated Parmesan cheese
1	tsp dried basil leaves
½	tsp garlic salt
½	c fat-free sour cream
2	Tbsp chopped fresh chives

1. Preheat the oven to 425°F. Pierce the potatoes a few times with a fork. Bake for 55 minutes, or until easily pierced with a fork. Remove from the oven, and let cool slightly.
2. Meanwhile, in a small bowl, combine the Parmesan, basil, and garlic salt.
3. When the potatoes are cool enough to handle, quarter them lengthwise. Scoop out the flesh, leaving a ¼"-thick shell. Reserve the flesh for another use. Cut the strips in half crosswise. You should have 24 wedges. Place on a baking sheet coated with cooking spray. Coat both sides of the potato wedges with cooking spray. Place skin side down on the sheet, and sprinkle with the Parmesan mixture.
4. Bake for 10 minutes, or until golden brown. To serve, top with dollops of sour cream. Sprinkle with the chives.

Makes 8 servings

Per serving: 73 cal, 4 g pro, 9 g carb, 2 g fat, 1 g sat. fat, 5 mg chol, 1 g fiber, 210 mg sodium
Diet exchanges: 0 milk, 0 vegetable, 0 fruit, ½ bread, ½ meat, 0 fat

Buffalo Chicken with Blue Cheese Dressing

Chicken drummettes have more meat than wings and can be easily skinned. When baked instead of fried, these nuggets are much lower in fat and calories.

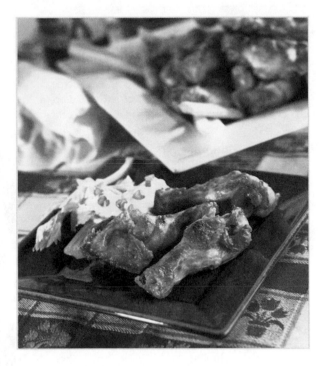

24	**chicken drummettes, skinned**
4	**Tbsp hot sauce**
2	**tsp vinegar**
¼	**tsp garlic powder**
⅓	**c crumbled blue cheese**
1	**c fat-free sour cream**
1	**scallion, chopped**
1	**Tbsp white wine vinegar**
1	**tsp sugar**
2	**lg ribs celery, cut into sticks**

1. Preheat the oven to 400°F. Coat a baking sheet with cooking spray.
2. In a large bowl, toss together the chicken, 2 tablespoons of the hot sauce, 1 teaspoon of the vinegar, and garlic powder. Arrange on the prepared baking sheet. Bake for 12 minutes, or until the juices run clear.
3. Meanwhile, in a medium bowl, combine the cheese, sour cream, scallion, vinegar, and sugar. Stir to mix, mashing the cheese with a spoon.
4. Remove the chicken from the oven. Drizzle with the remaining 2 tablespoons hot sauce and 1 teaspoon vinegar, tossing to mix. Serve with the blue cheese dressing and celery sticks.

Makes 24 servings

Per serving: 92 cal, 14 g pro, 2 g carb, 3 g fat, 1 g sat. fat, 50 mg chol, 0 g fiber, 99 mg sodium
Diet exchanges: 0 milk, 0 vegetable, 0 fruit, 0 bread, 2 meat, ½ fat

Orange Drop Cookies

Substituting reduced-fat cream cheese for some of the butter in baked goods such as these drop cookies cuts the calories while retaining the richness.

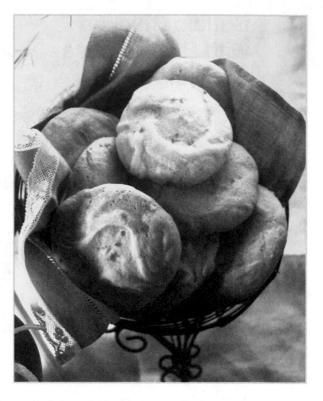

1⅓	c all-purpose flour
½	tsp baking powder
⅛	tsp baking soda
¼	tsp salt
¼	c butter, at room temperature
2	Tbsp reduced-fat cream cheese
1	egg
½	c sugar
1	Tbsp grated orange peel
1	tsp orange extract

1. Preheat the oven to 350°F. Line baking sheets with parchment.
2. In a medium bowl, combine the flour, baking powder, baking soda, and salt.
3. In a large bowl, with an electric mixer on medium speed, beat the butter, cream cheese, egg, sugar, orange peel, and orange extract for 3 minutes, or until light. The mixture will appear curdled. Beat in the flour mixture, a little at a time, until well blended.
4. Drop the batter by teaspoonfuls about 2 inches apart onto the prepared baking sheets. Bake for 10 minutes, or until the edges are golden. Remove, with the parchment, to a rack. Let cool for 10 minutes, and peel off the parchment. Repeat.

Makes 30 cookies

Per cookie: 53 cal, 1 g pro, 7 g carb, 2 g fat, 1 g sat. fat, 12 mg chol, 0 g fiber, 53 mg sodium
Diet exchanges: 0 milk, 0 vegetable, 0 fruit, ½ bread, 0 meat, ½ fat

Almond Macaroons

Healthy almonds are the basis of these crispy cookies. For more variety, try substituting hazelnuts.

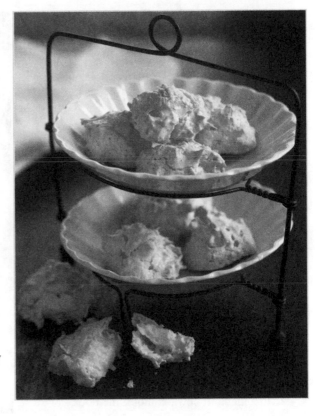

1½	c ground toasted almonds
¼	c all-purpose flour
¼	tsp salt
3	egg whites
½	tsp almond extract
1	c sugar

1. Preheat the oven to 325°F. Line baking sheets with parchment.
2. In a small bowl, combine the almonds, flour, and salt.
3. In a large bowl, with an electric mixer on high speed, beat the egg whites until soft peaks form. Add the almond extract. Gradually beat in the sugar, ¼ cup at a time, until stiff peaks form.
4. Fold the almond mixture into the egg whites.
5. Drop the batter by heaping teaspoonfuls 2 inches apart onto the prepared baking sheets.
6. Bake for 14 minutes, or until light brown. Remove, with the parchment, to a rack. Let cool for 10 minutes, and peel off the parchment. Repeat.

Makes 36 cookies

Per cookie: 56 cal, 2 g pro, 7 g carb, 3 g fat, 0 g sat. fat, 0 mg chol, 1 g fiber, 21 mg sodium
Diet exchanges: 0 milk, 0 vegetable, 0 fruit, ½ bread, 0 meat, ½ fat

Low-Fat Fudgy Brownies

Applesauce takes the place of some of the fat and sugar in this healthier version of a favorite chocolate goody.

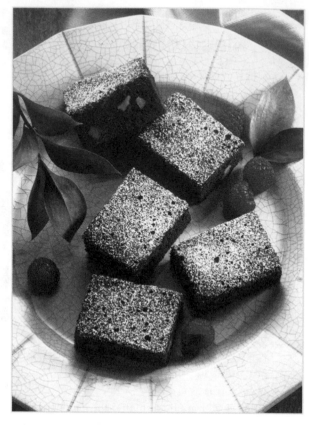

½	**c unbleached flour**
¾	**c cocoa powder**
½	**tsp baking powder**
¼	**tsp salt**
3	**egg whites**
2	**eggs, lightly beaten**
1	**c granulated sugar**
½	**c packed brown sugar**
⅔	**c unsweetened applesauce**
2	**tsp vanilla extract**
½	**c coarsely chopped walnuts**
	Confectioners' sugar

1. Preheat the oven to 350°F. Coat a 13" x 9" baking pan with cooking spray.
2. In a medium bowl, combine the flour, cocoa powder, baking powder, and salt.
3. In a large bowl, with an electric mixer on low speed, beat the egg whites until foamy. Gently stir in the eggs, granulated sugar, and brown sugar until well combined. Blend in the applesauce and vanilla extract. Stir in the flour mixture. Stir in the walnuts.
4. Spread into the prepared pan. Bake for 20 minutes, or until a wooden pick inserted in the center comes out clean. Do not overbake. Cool in the pan on a rack. Dust the confectioners' sugar over the brownies.

Makes 32 brownies

Per brownie: 70 cal, 2 g pro, 13 g carb, 2 g fat, 0 g sat. fat, 13 mg chol, 1 g fiber, 35 mg sodium
Diet exchanges: 0 milk, 0 vegetable, 0 fruit, ½ bread, 0 meat, ½ fat

‖ Mocha Frappé

Making coffee ice cubes adds body to this drink while keeping it fat-free.

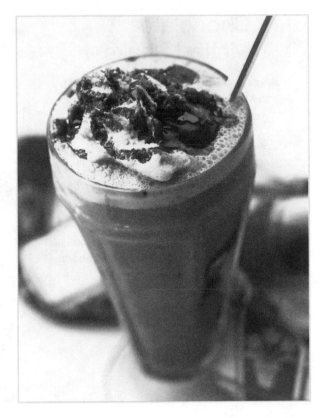

½	**c boiling water**
2	**tsp instant espresso powder**
2	**c fat-free milk**
3	**Tbsp fat-free chocolate syrup**
1	**c crushed ice**

1. In a measuring cup or bowl, combine the water and espresso powder. Stir to dissolve. Pour into an ice cube tray. Freeze for 2 hours, or until solid.
2. In a blender, combine the milk, chocolate syrup, and frozen coffee ice cubes. Blend until smooth. Add the ice, and blend until smooth.

Makes 2 servings

Per serving: 132 cal, 10 g pro, 22 g carb, 0 g fat, 0 g sat. fat, 5 mg chol, 1 g fiber, 168 mg sodium
Diet exchanges: 1 milk, 0 vegetable, 0 fruit, ½ bread, 0 meat, 0 fat

Chocolate Malted Shake

Fat-free milk and frozen yogurt combine with crushed ice to keep the calories to a minimum in this refreshing treat.

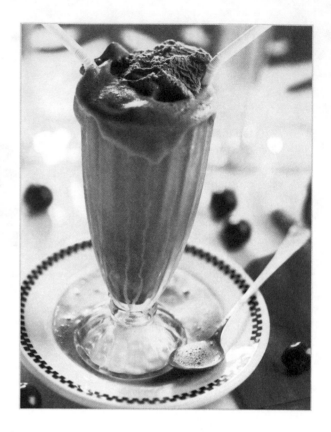

1½	**c fat-free frozen chocolate yogurt**
½	**c fat-free milk**
4½	**Tbsp chocolate malted milk powder**
1½	**c crushed ice**

1. In a blender, combine the yogurt, milk, and malted milk powder. Blend until smooth.

2. Add the ice, and blend until smooth.

Makes 2 servings

Per serving: 178 cal, 7 g pro, 39 g carb, 2 g fat, 1 g sat. fat, 3 mg chol, 1 g fiber, 122 mg sodium
Diet exchanges: ½ milk, 0 vegetable, 0 fruit, 2½ bread, 0 meat, 0 fat

Diabetes Information Sources

A guide to finding reliable diabetes information

American Diabetes Association (ADA)

1701 North Beauregard St.

Alexandria, VA 22311

Phone: (800) DIABETES (342-2383) or (703) 549-1500

Fax: (703) 549-6995

Web site: www.diabetes.org

To order ADA publications, contact the ADA Order Fulfillment Department, P.O. Box 930850,

Atlanta, GA 31193-0850, call (800) 232-6733, or visit their Web site.

Centers for Disease Control and Prevention (CDC)

Division of Diabetes Translation

P.O. Box 8728

Silver Spring, MD 20910

Phone: (877) CDC-DIAB (232-3422)

Fax: (301) 562-1050

E-mail: diabetes@cdc.gov

Web site: www.cdc.gov/diabetes

The CDC Web site includes fact sheets, statistics, publications, and information about

state diabetes control programs.

continued on p. 176

Diabetes Information Sources

Joslin Diabetes Center

One Joslin Place
Boston, MA 02215
Phone: (800) JOSLIN-1 (567-5461) or (617) 732-2400
Web site: www.joslin.org
Joslin Diabetes Center publishes books, videotapes, and other educational materials for people
with diabetes and for professionals. The center also publishes *Joslin*, a quarterly newsletter.

Juvenile Diabetes Research Foundation International (JDRF)

120 Wall St.
New York, NY 10005
Phone: (800) JDF-CURE (533-2873) or (212) 785-9500
Fax: (212) 785-9595
E-mail: info@jdfcure.org
Web site: www.jdf.org
JDRF publishes the quarterly journal *Countdown*, the quarterly newsletter *Research News*,
and a series of patient education brochures about type 1 and type 2 diabetes.

National Diabetes Information Clearinghouse (NDIC)

One Information Way
Bethesda, MD 20892-3560
Phone: (800) 860-8747 or (301) 654-3327
Fax: (301) 907-8906
E-mail: ndic@info.niddk.nih.gov
Web site: www.niddk.nih.gov
Diabetes education materials are available free or for a small fee. Literature searches on
myriad subjects related to diabetes are provided. NDIC also publishes *Diabetes Dateline*,
a quarterly newsletter for health professionals.

Diabetes Care Checklist

Take care of your health with these recommendations from the American Diabetes Association

	ADA Recommendations	Your Goal	Your Results	Date
AT EVERY DIABETES CHECKUP				
Check blood sugar:				
Before meals	80–120			
Before bed	100–140			
Check blood pressure	130/85			
Review meal plan	——			
Review activity level	——			
Check weight	——			
AT LEAST EVERY 6 MONTHS				
Check hemoglobin A1C	Below 7			
AT LEAST ONCE A YEAR				
Physical exam	——			
Complete foot exam	——			
Dilated eye exam	——			
Check microalbumin	Below 30			
Check cholesterol:				
Total	Below 200			
HDL	Above 45			
LDL	Below 100			
Check triglycerides	Below 200			
Flu shot	——			

Ask your doctor about getting a pneumonia shot. Report any unusual symptoms to your doctor.

The *Outsmart Diabetes* Food Shopping List

Have the right foods on hand to make healthy eating a snap

Fruit

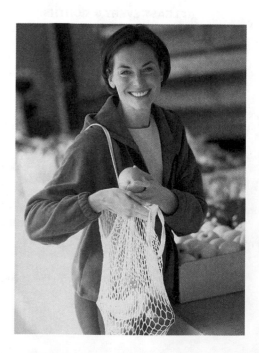

Apples
Apricots
Bananas
Blueberries
Cantaloupe
Cherries
Grapefruit
Guava
Kiwifruit
Mango
Oranges
Papaya
Passion fruit
Pineapple
Plums
Seedless grapes

Vegetables

Baby carrots
Broccoli
Brussels sprouts
Cabbage
Cauliflower
Escarole
Fennel
Jicama
Kale
Onions
Plantains
Potatoes
Pumpkin
Red bell peppers
Spinach
Squash
Sweet potatoes
Tomatoes (including cherry and grape)

Dried Fruit

Apricots
Cherries
Cranberries
Peaches
Prunes
Raisins

Frozen Fruit

Blueberries
Pineapple chunks
Raspberries
Strawberries

Meats

Lean top round beef
Pork tenderloin
Skinless chicken
Turkey breast

Seafood

Cod
Haddock
Mackerel
Salmon
Snapper
Sole
Tuna

Vegetarian Burgers

Breads

Oat bran
Pita
Tortillas
Whole wheat breads
  and rolls

Grains and Legumes

Barley
Brown rice
Bulgur
Couscous
Dried peas
Lentils
Whole wheat pasta

BEANS, DRIED OR CANNED

Black
Chickpeas
Kidney
Lima
Navy
White

Oils and Condiments

OILS

Canola
Olive
Toasted sesame

CONDIMENTS

Anchovy paste
Balsamic vinegar
Fat-free mayonnaise
Horseradish
Hot peppers
Mustard
Onion paste
Sun-dried tomato paste
Wasabi paste

Herbs and Spices

Garlic

DRIED

Basil
Dill
Oregano
Rosemary
Thyme

GROUND OR WHOLE

Black peppercorn
Chili powder
Cinnamon
Cumin
Curry powder
Garlic powder
Ginger
Ground red pepper
Paprika
Red-pepper flakes

Canned Goods

Fat-free chicken broth
Mandarin oranges
Pineapple chunks
Salsa
Soup (not cream-based
  varieties)
Water-packed tuna

Dairy and Eggs

Cheddar cheese

Cottage cheese

Eggs and egg whites

Fat-free milk

Fat-free yogurt

Feta cheese

Grated cheese

Low-fat or fat-free sour cream

Low-fat mozzarella

Ricotta cheese

String cheese

Drinks

**100% FRUIT JUICES
AND NECTARS**

Apple

Apricot

Grape

Orange

Papaya

Peach

Pear

OTHER DRINKS

Green tea

Seltzer

Sparkling water

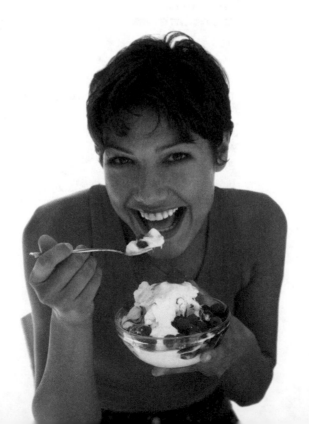

Text Credits

Part 2, Chapter 5: Trace Minerals That Make a Difference
Reprinted from *Prevention's New Foods for Healing* by Selene Yeager and the Editors of Prevention Health Books © 1998 by Rodale Press.

Part 3, Chapters 6 and 10
Reprinted from *Prevention's Healthy Cooking: Eat Up, Slim Down* by Jane Kirby, RD, and David Joachim © 2001 by Rodale Inc.

Part 3, Chapter 8
Reprinted from *Healthy Homestyle Cooking* © 1994 by Evelyn Tribole.

Part 4, Chapter 12
Reprinted from *Prevention's Complete Book of Walking* by Maggie Spilner © 2000 by Rodale Inc.

Part 6
Recipes reprinted from: *Rodale's New Classics: Cookies, Brownies, Muffins & More* by Anne Egan © 2000 by Rodale Inc., *Rodale's New Classics: Decadent Desserts* by Anne Egan © 2001 by Rodale Inc., *Rodale's New Classics: Savory Soups & Stews* by Anne Egan © 2000 by Rodale Inc., *Rodale's New Classics Cookbook: Family Favorites* © 1999 by Rodale Inc., *Prevention Magazine's Quick & Healthy Low-Fat Cooking: Fabulous No-Guilt Desserts* © 1996 by Rodale Press, *Prevention Magazine's Quick & Healthy Home Cooking* © 1995 by Rodale Press, *Jeanne Jones' Homestyle Cooking Made Healthy* © 1999 by Jeanne Jones, *Prevention's Quick & Healthy Family Favorites Cookbook* © 2000 by Rodale Inc., *Healthy Homestyle Cooking* © 1994 by Evelyn Tribole, *Prevention's Healthy Cooking: Eat Up, Slim Down* by Jane Kirby, RD, and David Joachim © 2001 by Rodale Inc.

Photo and Illustration Credits

Subject Index

Underscored page references indicate sidebars and tables.

A

Abdominal circumference, measuring, <u>81</u>
Abdominal fat
  calculating, from abdominal circumference, <u>81</u>
  charting reduction of, <u>83</u>
  health risks from, <u>4</u>, 79, 80
  steps for reducing, 80–83
Acarbose, as oral diabetes medication, 14
Accu-Chek D-Tector, for diagnosing diabetes, <u>8</u>
Acetazolamide, as oral diabetes medication, 12–13
Alcohol
  abdominal fat from, 83
  in Diabetes-Blocking Diet, 35
  as occasional treat, <u>59</u>
Alpha-glycosides inhibitors, as oral diabetes
      medication, 14
Alpha-lipoic acid, for diabetic neuropathy, 100–101,
      <u>100</u>
American Diabetes Association, 175
Apligraf, for foot ulcers, <u>95</u>
Aspirin, for preventing heart disease, 98
Avia 362 shoe, for fitness walks, 77

B

Baking, as low-fat cooking method, <u>55</u>
Beans, for reducing diabetes risk, 31
Belly fat. *See* Abdominal fat
Biguanide, as oral diabetes medication, 14
Bladder infections, preventing, 96–97
Blood glucose monitor, 16–17
Blood sugar
  controlling
    with meal planning, <u>41</u>
    with minerals, <u>35</u>
    for preventing bladder infections, 97
    for preventing gum disease, 94
    for preventing vision problems, 93
  function of, 3
  high vs. low, 8
  interpreting test scores of, 7
  monitoring, 15
    devices for, 16–17, 19
    after dining out, 61
    before exercise, 69
    with hemoglobin A1c test, <u>18</u>
  postmeal spikes in, <u>97</u>
  uncontrolled, immediate problems from, 7–8
  how walking affects, 72–73
Body mass index, how to calculate, <u>24</u>
Bone building, from strength training, 86
Brain, effect of exercise on, 71
Bread, exchange servings of, 40
Breakfast, importance of, 64
Buddies, workout, 83, <u>86</u>

C

Caffeine, for boosting metabolism, 86
Calcium-rich foods, for reducing diabetes risk,
    30–31
Calcium supplements, for reducing diabetes risk,
    33
Calorie-burning
  metabolism and, 84, 85
  from strength training, 86
Calorie counting, vs. fat restriction, 64
Calorie needs
  calculating, <u>39</u>
  exchange allowance for, <u>40</u>
Carbohydrates
  controlling, for blood sugar balance, <u>41</u>
  counting, 44
  glycemic index of, 46–47
Casual walks, shoes for, 77–78
Causes of diabetes, <u>4</u>
Centers for Disease Control and Prevention, 175
Chair dip, in strength training workout, <u>89</u>
Checklist, diabetes care, 177
Chest press, in strength training workout, <u>89</u>

Recipe Index

Boldface page references indicate photographs.

Conversion Chart

These equivalents have been slightly rounded to make measuring easier.

VOLUME MEASUREMENTS

US	Imperial	Metric
¼ tsp	–	1 ml
½ tsp	–	2 ml
1 tsp	–	5 ml
1 Tbsp	–	15 ml
2 Tbsp (1 oz)	1 fl oz	30 ml
¼ cup (2 oz)	2 fl oz	60 ml
⅓ cup (3 oz)	3 fl oz	80 ml
½ cup (4 oz)	4 fl oz	120 ml
⅔ cup (5 oz)	5 fl oz	160 ml
¾ cup (6 oz)	6 fl oz	180 ml
1 cup (8 oz)	8 fl oz	240 ml

WEIGHT MEASUREMENTS

US	Metric
1 oz	30 g
2 oz	60 g
4 oz (¼ lb)	115 g
5 oz (⅓ lb)	145 g
6 oz	170 g
7 oz	200 g
8 oz (½ lb)	230 g
10 oz	285 g
12 oz (¾ lb)	340 g
14 oz	400 g
16 oz (1 lb)	455 g
2.2 lb	1 kg

LENGTH MEASUREMENTS

US	Metric
¼"	0.6 cm
½"	1.25 cm
1"	2.5 cm
2"	5 cm
4"	11 cm
6"	15 cm
8"	20 cm
10"	25 cm
12" (1')	30 cm

PAN SIZES

US	Metric
8" cake pan	20 × 4 cm sandwich or cake tin
9" cake pan	23 × 3.5 cm sandwich or cake tin
11" × 7" baking pan	28 × 18 cm baking tin
13" × 9" baking pan	32.5 × 23 cm baking tin
15" × 10" baking pan	38 × 25.5 cm baking tin (Swiss roll tin)
1½ qt baking dish	1.5 liter baking dish
2 qt baking dish	2 liter baking dish
2 qt rectangular baking dish	30 × 19 cm baking dish
9" pie plate	22 × 4 or 23 × 4 cm pie plate
7" or 8" springform pan	18 or 20 cm springform or loose-bottom cake tin
9" × 5" loaf pan	23 × 13 cm or 2 lb narrow loaf tin or pâté tin

TEMPERATURES

Fahrenheit	Centigrade	Gas
140°	60°	–
160°	70°	–
180°	80°	–
225°	105°	¼
250°	120°	½
275°	135°	1
300°	150°	2
325°	160°	3
350°	180°	4
375°	190°	5
400°	200°	6
425°	220°	7
450°	230°	8
475°	245°	9
500°	260°	–